LEADING THROUGH A PANDEMIC

LEADING THROUGH A PANDEMIC

THE INSIDE STORY OF HUMANITY, INNOVATION, AND LESSONS LEARNED DURING THE COVID-19 CRISIS

MICHAEL J. DOWLING
AND
CHARLES KENNEY

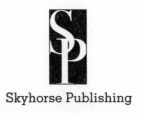

Skyhorse Publishing

Skyhorse Publishing books may be purchased in bulk at special discounts for sales promotion, corporate gifts, fund-raising, or educational purposes. Special editions can also be created to specifications. For details, contact the Special Sales Department, Skyhorse Publishing, 307 West 36th Street, 11th Floor, New York, NY 10018 or info@skyhorsepublishing.com.

Skyhorse® and Skyhorse Publishing® are registered trademarks of Skyhorse Publishing, Inc.®, a Delaware corporation.

Visit our website at www.skyhorsepublishing.com.

10 9 8 7 6 5 4 3 2 1

Library of Congress Cataloging-in-Publication Data is available on file.

Cover design by Brian Peterson
Pictured on the cover: Nina Corsini, physical therapist, Northwell Health Glen Cove Hospital

Print ISBN: 978-1-5107-6384-5
Ebook ISBN: 978-1-5107-6385-2

Printed in the United States of America

We dedicate this book to our Northwell colleagues for their life saving work—to the nurses, doctors, respiratory therapists, pharmacists, house-keepers, food service workers, EMTs and paramedics, physical therapists, researchers, transporters, social workers, security staff, and all of the other men and women whose work saved countless lives.

Contents

Report from the Front

Emily Fawcett, RN

I took care of a veteran on the palliative care unit of a COVID floor at Lenox Hill Hospital in Manhattan. He was in his seventies, dying from COVID. His children wanted to come in and say goodbye to their dad. Since the pandemic, we've been very strict on visitors, but if somebody is actively dying, we try to accommodate the family, so we arranged for them to come in and say goodbye. Our nurse manager, Renee Sanchez, whose dad is also a vet, said we had to do something for this family. The children came in and we all geared up in our personal protective equipment (PPE) and went into the room, too. They were extremely proud of their father and his service to our country.

The son and daughter both spoke about their dad. A vet who works in our hospital, Frank Kachelle, said a few words of appreciation. Deirdre O'Flaherty, our director of nursing, found the US Navy band's version of "The Star Spangled Banner" and she played it on her iPhone. Deirdre's husband is also a vet.

The children were emotional, but they had this beautiful moment, which so many people didn't have during COVID. A lot of people have died alone. I think this family at least had their peace. They got to say goodbye, and we cried with them.

* * *

Around that same time I was taking care of a lady in her seventies whose husband was very sick. I really got to know her. I had met her in the emergency room the week before because her husband had come in very, very sick from COVID and had to be put on a ventilator in the ICU.

I'm a float nurse, so I work everywhere in the hospital, which gave me a very good perspective during this whole thing, because I saw it from the lens of the emergency room. I saw it from the lens of being on the actively dying COVID floor. I saw it from the lens of being in the critical care stepdown unit trying to save people. I kind of got a full spectrum of treating COVID patients.

A few days after her husband was admitted, this lady became sick also. She was very vibrant, very young for her age. She was on oxygen and definitely sick, but not as sick as her husband. I was taking care of her on a unit that was the next hallway over from the ICU where her husband was, but she couldn't see him, couldn't be there with him. She couldn't hold his hand or touch his face. All she could do to feel connected to him was to pray for him. At night I would be with her and we would pray. She was lovely. She was extremely sick herself, and yet she was so nice to me. We cried together, we held hands together. I was pretty tough on her. I made her get out of the bed and sit in the chair, and she was huffing and puffing. She wasn't eating, so I made her eat. Every day when I walked in she was like, *Emily!*

Her husband was on a ventilator for multiple weeks. I thought he had no chance of living. He was extremely, extremely sick to the point where his wife and I had a conversation about who would make final medical decisions. They had no children so we had to call one of their relatives to make him the health-care proxy in the event that, God forbid, if anything happened to both of them there would be a proxy to make their medical decisions. That was really hard. I felt really close to her. I actually thought her husband would not make it, but then he got the breathing tube out and came off the ventilator. This was when a majority of patients on ventilators did not make it. But he started to recover.

I showed up for a shift after a few days off and there they were together, she and her husband recovering in the same room. Before I even walked in the room she heard my voice and she said to her husband, *oh my God, it's my nurse Emily. This is one who took care of me.*

And I loved meeting him and telling him how I had been taking care of his wife and how we had prayed for him. I will never forget that couple. They ended up going home together.

* * *

At the beginning there was so much anxiety. Would we run out of ventilators? Would we have to choose who got a ventilator? What was that going to look like? And then when we were at the top of the curve, I was just working, working, working, too busy to think about anything. Coming off the curve was very weird. You'd just gone through this crazy thing. I had no time to process it. I was running on adrenaline, running on anxiety.

I've been a nurse for almost ten years. I have never in my ten years done an overtime shift. I always thought I was a better nurse when I had some time off and would come in refreshed. So the nursing office said *Emily, are you okay? Why are you working so much?* I just felt this great need to be on the front line for my city. I wanted to be in the thick of things. I felt better being at work than being home in my apartment alone. I wasn't sleeping. I wasn't eating. I lost a lot of weight.

I wanted to be there for New Yorkers. I wanted to fight COVID for New York. I wanted to defend my city against this weird virus that we knew nothing about. So I felt this calling. I've done a lot of mission work, a lot of mission trips internationally—Kenya, Venezuela, and for the hurricane in Puerto Rico. I'd worked aboard the USNS *Comfort*. I felt like I was on a mission for New York City. I lived at the hospital for that month and a half, and it was just where I needed to be.

Introduction

Humbling Lessons

At Northwell Health, we started preparing for the coronavirus pandemic twenty-two years before it arrived in New York. In 1998, FBI Special Agent John O'Neill, head of the Joint Terrorism Task Force, told one of our senior executives, Northwell's Executive Vice President Kathleen Gallo, that he expected an attack on the city. In that conversation, Special Agent O'Neill expressed frustration. He said he had talked with people from various hospital systems, but that no one seemed to take him seriously. He told Gallo that he did not know when, where, or how exactly, but that he was convinced some kind of attack was coming. State-sponsored terrorism was happening more frequently, and non-state actors were growing in numbers and sophistication.

Gallo was struck by the depth of the agent's knowledge and the intensity of his conviction. Their meeting led to decisions at Northwell that would forever change our system's culture and capabilities. Energized by what O'Neill told us, we hosted a conference on weapons of mass destruction to which we invited major health systems in New York. Most weren't interested. O'Neill was scheduled to speak but was called to Yemen to investigate a terrorist attack on a Navy ship. He sent a colleague to fill in for him at our conference and, remarkably enough, O'Neill's colleague displayed a large photograph of a man no one in the room had ever heard of—Osama Bin Laden. The agent said that this man could potentially attack New York. Tragically, after O'Neill retired from the FBI, he took a position as head of security for the World Trade Center in New York and was killed in the 9/11 attack. And here we are in 2020 with the coronavirus as the newest weapon of mass destruction.

As we discussed the inevitability of terrorism and the need to prepare two decades ago, it was clear that many other types of emergencies could be headed our way as well. We made a decision to build a robust emergency preparedness infrastructure within our health system based on a simple assumption: *Bad things will happen. We have to be ready.* But what bad things? Terrorist attacks, as the agent suggested. Also major weather events, utility outages, cyber threats, and the potential for infectious disease outbreaks, which have always been near the top of our threat list. We had to be ready for anything and everything. We set about making emergency preparedness a major capability within our growing health system, and toward that end we established a network incident command structure of a kind widely relied upon by military and law enforcement organizations. It is known as an *all-hazards* approach, on the theory that it prepares the organization for any type of disaster and involves the creation of an emergency leadership unit able to deploy personnel and resources from every part of the organization to wherever they are needed. We hired and promoted experienced emergency management experts, invested millions of dollars in equipment, and trained thousands of staff members. Creating this type of capability was unusual for a health-care system in part because it required a major financial investment with zero anticipated return on investment (ROI). A significant disaster response capability was considered the job of governments—federal, state, county, or municipal—and rarely the role of private health systems. But we believed that our emergency capability would one day save lives. And that is what it did during the coronavirus pandemic.

* * *

At Northwell, we took care of more COVID-19 patients than any other health system in the United States. We nearly doubled our capacity of three thousand beds in a matter of weeks and that was barely enough. Our frontline workers saw illness and death on a scale none had ever witnessed before. The pandemic stands, without doubt, as the most frightening, overwhelming experience any of us have ever been through.

And the most humbling. We were stunned by the power of the virus and the disease it caused.

As we reflected upon the experience we sought to identify lessons learned to help us, as well as others in health care and government, prepare for next time. Some of what we believed before the crisis was confirmed. Bad things will happen—of this there is no doubt—and in order to care for patients, our absolute number one priority must be protecting the physical and emotional health of our staff, as well as ensuring their safety.

We also reaffirmed our belief that an emergency management capability should be a core competence of every health system. Preparation rests upon creating a culture where emergency teams are valued and respected throughout the organization, and where emergency management departments are as essential to the organization as departments of cardiology or oncology. This is far from the reality at most health systems in the United States today and one of the more dangerous holes in the country's overall medical capability.

We learned that an emergency preparedness culture gives leaders the confidence to change and improve in the midst of chaos. Crisis situations are illuminating and, quite often, good ideas and improved processes emerge.

Our long-held belief in the efficacy of an incident command structure similar to what is used in the military and by first responders was confirmed. This simplified chain of command enabled us to make crucial decisions faster than ever.

We learned that the importance of relationships with vendors is magnified in a crisis and that vendor relationships nurtured over time prove far more durable than purely transactional relationships.

We learned how to expand our inpatient capacity far beyond what we had ever believed possible.

We learned the remarkable morale-boosting power of leaders going to the front lines to be present with the troops, to support them and to try in some way to help calm their fears.

We learned that low-income and minority neighborhoods were particularly vulnerable to the virus, further highlighting persistent inequities in access to care and health outcomes.

We learned the power of an integrated health system. In the pandemic crisis, the scale, adaptability, and integrated nature of our organization saved lives. Large, integrated medical systems have been much maligned in recent years, but after this experience that attitude may soften.

We learned that by integrating research into the emergency response we could perform clinical trials even during a crisis, producing data to benefit the entire world.

We learned that acceptance of telehealth by patients and providers is growing because of its convenience and effectiveness.

We learned—or, rather, our belief was reaffirmed—that the major insurance companies are more interested in profits than people's health.

We learned that stripped-down regulations gave us invaluable flexibility to perform quickly and effectively, that we can handle a major crisis and not buckle under its assault, and that we can collaborate well with competing health systems.

We learned what real leadership looked like—Governor Andrew Cuomo's calm, fact-based approach.

Our belief that politics has no place in the world of science was reaffirmed.

We learned what it was like to be in the epicenter of a global pandemic—learned firsthand how to care for 16,655 COVID inpatients while we treated and released 10,465 patients in our emergency departments, cared for 20,506 in our ambulatory centers and 2,231 in our post-acute locations—a grand total of 49,857 COVID-19-positive patients. Tragically, we lost twenty of our beloved fellow Northwell employees to the virus. (Numbers as of July 1, 2020.)

And when there was a resurgence of the virus in parts of the country during the early summer, we were reminded of the harsh reality that the coronavirus will be with us for at least the foreseeable future.

* * *

At Northwell, we had advantages going into the crisis. One was our size—twenty-three hospitals in the Greater New York area, eight hundred ambulatory sites, post-acute services, medical and nursing schools, a major institute for medical research, a core testing laboratory, nursing homes and home care, as well as a centrally organized transport system with a fleet of ambulances that allows us to move patients quickly and safely.

As valuable as our size proved to be, our emergency preparedness culture—developed in the years since Agent O'Neill issued his warning to us—proved even more important to our ability to deal with the crisis. Any hospital or health system, no matter its size, can also aspire to a culture of preparedness, and we should all be working together on developing this culture within all systems. In the time ahead, working with Governor Cuomo and leaders of other health systems, we will no doubt identify important steps that need to be taken in this process. But before we do anything collaboratively, there are two changes that are foundational:

- First, every hospital and health system, large and small, must develop a core capability in emergency management. This requires having the equipment and personnel necessary to manage any and all emergencies from hurricanes to pandemics. Government financial support will be required for many organizations to accomplish this.
- Second, every hospital and health system, large and small, must do the hard work of creating a culture in which an emergency capability is valued and respected throughout the organization. Few organizations in the United States have achieved this level of practical and cultural readiness.

We learned that, in training to prepare for a disaster, you know you are ready when your organization is, in the words of one of our emergency management leaders, "comfortable being uncomfortable" in a crisis. It would be a mistake to believe that only large systems can be prepared. Health-care entities of various sizes can certainly achieve an increased level of practical and cultural readiness. And given all that can go wrong in the twenty-first century—in the New York area in particular with hurricanes, blackouts, terrorism, pandemics, etc.—there is a responsibility to do so. We believe that practical and cultural readiness are prerequisites to the ability of health-care professionals throughout the United

States to coordinate efforts—with other entities, with state and local governments, with first responders—so that no one is overwhelmed and all patients are properly cared for.

* * *

The biggest story of the pandemic is the speed and lethality of the contagion. The next biggest story is the courage and professionalism of those who fought it on the front lines. Consider this scene that staff members faced each day, described by Dr. Lawrence Smith, Northwell physician in chief and dean of the Donald and Barbara Zucker School of Medicine:

> In the hospital it is a very sad, stressful environment—almost surreal. I've been practicing medicine for a long time and I have never been in a hospital where [so many] patients are on ventilators completely sedated, completely paralyzed, not moving a muscle. Not a visitor in the entire hospital. Bodies lying bed to bed to bed, and the only noise in the room is the hum of the ventilators. And these patients never speak, never move, and yet they are all potential killers of the staff because they're all shedding virus. I've been in ICUs and hospital wards for forty years now. I've never seen what the inside of Long Island Jewish Hospital looks like right now, with just endless rows of bodies that are alive, but they don't move and there's nobody there to tell you about them. The staff has never heard these people even speak in most cases because the speaking ended when they arrived in the emergency room. It's surreal. It's frightening.

In normal times, when doctors and nurses report for work, they have little fear of being harmed, but in this crisis, they lived with fear, especially early on. Not only doctors and nurses but physician assistants, nurse practitioners, respiratory therapists—including pregnant mothers and many people caring for children or sick parents at home—still answered the call. They lived with the fear that they could get sick or even die, that they might infect a loved one. Some people simply couldn't handle it or felt that working would be too great a risk for vulnerable family members, so they went on leave from work. But the overwhelming majority of our people managed the fear. Many got sick, but most recovered and returned to work.

In the modern age the term "hero" has been much overused. True heroism is a rare and beautiful thing. Merriam-Webster's dictionary defines a hero as "a mythological or legendary figure often of divine descent endowed with great strength or ability; an illustrious warrior; a person admired for achievements and noble qualities; one who shows great courage." This describes health-care workers in 2020. The physical challenge of caring for gravely ill patients is one thing. The psychological burden is quite another.

All frontline workers sacrificed their safety, and some gave their lives. These men and women, clad in scrubs, gowns, masks, and shields, made Hippocrates proud. They showed up, shift after shift, the pressure of fear in their chests, and cared for the gravely ill. They conveyed the final moments of loved ones' lives to family members via Zoom and FaceTime. They saw colleagues fall. They contracted the disease and died. As leaders, those of us in health care and government owe it to our frontline teams to do nothing less than scour this experience for lessons that will improve our future readiness. As Peggy Noonan put it in the *Wall Street Journal*: "The hidden gift of this pandemic is that this isn't the most terrible one, the next one or some other one down the road is. This is the one where we learn how to handle that coming pandemic."

Character reveals itself in crisis, and that was surely the case in the midst of the pandemic. Some hospitals and health-care workers prepared well and weathered the storm. Others, lacking preparation, were overwhelmed. In too much of America, a lack of preparedness was on stark display: doctors and nurses begging for masks, infected by those they treated. Thousands of patients died alone. Medical tents were set up in Central Park. A president claiming the situation was "totally under control" before more than one hundred thousand died.

* * *

In May 2020, after the virus had passed the peak in New York, Governor Cuomo announced the Reimagining New York venture to plan for the new reality in the post-COVID world. He enlisted one of us—Michael Dowling, CEO of Northwell—to lead the health-care part of that initiative. We hope the experiences and lessons we share in this book will help advance that initiative and that, in turn, others across our nation will learn from what we have been through. In this book, we will identify lessons that apply not only to our health system, but to all hospitals, whether individual stand-alone entities or larger systems. The lessons we've written about apply to both private not-for-profit hospital systems like our own and to public hospitals. The lessons, individually and collectively, will make clear the need for significant change throughout the health-care-delivery system if we are to be prepared for the next crisis, whatever it happens to be.

Each chapter of this book summarizes essential lessons learned and then tells the story or stories that reveal those lessons. Most importantly, we have synthesized the stories and lessons within the book and proposed a series of specific steps that health systems need to take in order to be ready for the next pandemic. This thirteen-point prescription is presented in the final chapter, with the hope that medical and public health professionals as well as government officials and the public will recognize that failing to take the prescribed steps will leave our nation vulnerable to a far more severe attack from the next virus.

CHAPTER ONE

Epicenter—The Peak of the Crisis

Lessons
- Staff demonstrates extraordinary courage, compassion, creativity, and resilience during crisis. They possess a natural desire to come together and succeed for the common good.
- Being part of a large, integrated system has enormous advantages.
- Load balancing—the ability to transport patients from overwhelmed facilities to other hospitals—saves lives. This requires a central transfer system.
- Don't prepare for the worst case. Instead, expect and prepare for a reality even worse than that.
- Assess the long-term impact on staff dealing with anxiety, fear and death.

If you were searching for the epicenter of the COVID-19 virus in the United States, you would have to make your way to the borough of Queens in New York City, more specifically to 102-01 66th Road in the Forest Hills neighborhood. There you would find Long Island Jewish Forest Hills Hospital, part of the Northwell Health system, where the virus unleashed its fury.

Queens County, with a population of 2.3 million people, is the most diverse in the United States. A total of 164 languages and dialects are spoken there. Our hospital, where the number one language is Spanish,

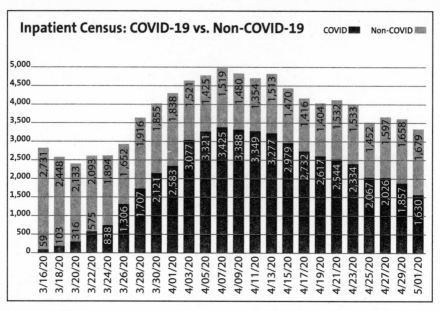

Northwell cared for all patients (COVID and non-COVID) throughout the course of the crisis. The peak was on April 7 at 3,425 COVID patients and approximately 5,000 in total.

followed quickly by Russian, is in the center of this diversity. Our immediate neighbors are largely Bukharian Jews who fled from Uzbekistan when the Soviet Union dissolved in the 1990s. Nearby neighborhoods such as Corona and Jackson Heights are predominantly Hispanic, while Jamaica and Richmond Hill are mostly African American, Caribbean, and Indian. In Flushing, there is a large Asian population, which is also growing in the area surrounding the hospital. The demography of this neighborhood made for a perfect storm—tight living quarters, many multigenerational households with not a lot of ability for people to self-isolate, pockets of low-income residents, and high reliance on public transportation.

At a hospital a ten-minute drive from Forest Hills Hospital, there was a dire warning of what was headed our way. A headline in the *New York Times* read: "13 Deaths in a Day: An 'Apocalyptic' Coronavirus Surge at a N.Y.C. Hospital." The story focused on our Queens neighbor, Elmhurst Hospital, which is not part of our Northwell system but rather of the New York City public hospital system. In the harrowing *Times* story, a doctor at Elmhurst was quoted as saying, "I don't have the support that I need, and even just the materials that I need, physically, to take care of my patients. . . . The anxiety of this situation is really overwhelming. . . .

We don't have the protective equipment that we should have. . . . I want people to know that this is bad. People are dying. We don't have the tools that we need in the emergency department and in the hospital to take care of them."* The *Times* reported that some patients at Elmhurst died in the emergency department awaiting treatment. Who would ever have believed that you would hear the words "apocalyptic" and "besieged" to describe the scene inside a hospital in a major American city?

* * *

During a leadership team meeting at our Forest Hills hospital in March, with the virus approaching, you could sense growing anxiety. The news from China and Italy was alarming. Team members engaged in emotionally charged arguments about what we should do. At this point Susan Browning, executive director of the hospital, interjected forcefully: "Guys, stop. We have a surge plan; we developed the surge plan when times were calm. We are going to take that surge plan out right now and we're going to talk from the surge plan. We are not going to make things up on the fly."

Forest Hills is one of Northwell's smaller hospitals, with an average daily census of about 150 medical patients; typically a bit higher in winter and lower in summer. With the expected influx of COVID-19 patients, the surge plan called for us to open up areas that normally would not be used for patient care. We refitted the endoscopy suite to accommodate fifteen new beds and emptied out a conference room and added ten beds. We moved half of our maternity patients from a new, state-of-the-art unit into triple-bedded rooms in an older part of our facility and added twenty additional medical beds to the vacated maternity unit. We converted our fourteen-bay preoperative ambulatory surgery area to fourteen inpatient beds. Our eight-bay post-anesthesia care unit accommodated eight more inpatient beds while, at the same time, we turned some medical floor beds into intensive care units. By the time the surge plan was executed, we had the capability to care for nearly seventy additional patients in every corner of the hospital.

---

* Michael Rothfeld, Somini Sengupta, Joseph Goldstein and Brian M. Rosenthal, "'People Are Dying': 72 Hours Inside a
   N.Y.C. Hospital Battling Coronavirus," *New York Times*, March 25, 2020.

And then came the onslaught, or tsunami, or whatever other metaphor you may choose for an overwhelming and unstoppable force: A deadly pathogen kicked down our doors and fought us for control of our hospital. As we said earlier, on an average day at Forest Hills, we see about 150 patients in our emergency department. At one point, there were 249 patients in our ED, 90 percent of them very sick COVID patients. Our emergency area got so crowded that if we had added one more body we would have been in violation of the New York City Fire Department occupancy codes. Forest Hills went from an eighteen-bed ICU with average daily occupancy of fourteen beds to three ICU units with a census reaching forty-nine; from a handful of ventilated patients in the building at any point to fifty patients on vents.

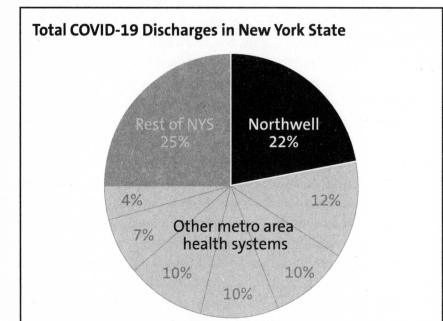

Total COVID-19 Discharges in New York State

Rest of NYS 25%

Northwell 22%

12%

4%

7%

Other metro area health systems

10%

10%

10%

We learned what it was like to be in the epicenter of a global pandemic; — learned firsthand how to care for 16,655 COVID inpatients while we treated and released 10,465 patients in our Emergency Departments, cared for 20,506 in our ambulatory centers and 2,231 in our post acute locations—a grand total of 49,857 COVID-19-positive patients.

By no means was Forest Hills the only one of our hospitals under siege. Most of our entities faced comparable surges in patients, including Long Island Jewish Medical Center in Queens, Long Island Jewish Valley Stream Hospital, North Shore University Hospital in Manhasset, and others. We were so inundated that we would wind up treating a full 20 percent of all COVID patients in the state of New York, more than anyone else.

The average ED patients we were accustomed to seeing were people with broken bones, cardiac issues, and a wide assortment of other mostly non-life-threatening conditions. The COVID patients were much sicker. COVID was different, and sometimes possessed a stealthy quality. The virus seemed to hide, holding back its full force and then suddenly unleashing it in a horrific assault on a patient's system. Many people presented at Forest Hills with relatively mild flu-like symptoms; not feeling well but not sick enough to be admitted to the hospital. Many of these patients went home and rode out their illness. But then there were others who, after being sent home to recover, would return just days later. With some of them it seemed as though a viral bomb had detonated within their bodies, generating fevers, chest pressure, and persistent headaches. Patients gasped for air. Shockingly rapid deterioration followed, with patients needing to be intubated and placed on ventilators, where the prognosis was grim.

"We were seeing sickness unlike any that we had seen," said Susan Browning. "These patients were just so sick, and they would decompensate so quickly, so you could literally be talking with a patient and an hour later, the patient could be coding"—that is, suffering a life-threatening condition such as a heart attack. For all our planning, for all of our culture of emergency preparation, in only a matter of days we exceeded the highest numbers we had ever envisioned in our surge plan at Forest Hills. Those admitted remained for double the length of stay of patients in normal times. We were doubling the percentage of emergency department patients admitted to the hospital and doubling their length of stay on top of that.

And then on a particular Saturday night in March, all hell broke loose. Dr. Thomas McGinn, deputy physician-in-chief at Northwell, received an urgent call for more staff at Forest Hills. "It was not just a stress on our overall system," he recalled, "it was a major assault." And in that assault, our staff at Forest Hills was pushed to the brink. Normally, in our Forest Hills ICU, a nurse would care for one or two patients; during the crisis our ICU nurses cared for as many as five patients. Normally at Forest Hills you hear urgent rapid response calls a half dozen times in twenty-four hours; now the calls were coming every ten minutes, hour after hour. Staff members were shell shocked. Nothing like this had ever happened before in our hospital. On a typical day before COVID changed the world, Forest Hills might have one patient die. In one twenty-four-hour period in March 2020, the virus took the lives of seventeen souls in our hospital.

* * *

Dr. Teresa Amato, head of emergency services at Forest Hills Hospital, felt a strong connection to the other sixteen emergency departments throughout the Northwell system. She knew her counterparts well and had joined in regular meetings with them where the ED nurses and physician leaders would share ideas for implementing best practices. If something innovative can work in one ED, we thought, let's see whether we can make it work in others as well. There was a sense of mission and camaraderie among this group of emergency specialists. "We had our individual needs and concerns, but at the end of the day, whatever we did, we kind of did it all together as a service line," she said. The emergency departments also shared a very good IT structure, with a dashboard that enabled any of the leaders to see immediately what the situation was across the system: how many patients were being held in EDs and where exactly, how long the wait was, how many had been admitted, where there were open beds, and so on. We looked at our emergency capacity as a whole system, not just individual hospitals or individual ambulatory sites. That was the infrastructure in place when, as Amato put it, the virus struck and "each day got worse and worse." It was very soon clear that she was at the epicenter of the outbreak. In an ideal world, before transporting very sick patients—and especially ICU patients—it is preferable to send additional staff in to care for them. And that is what happened initially at Forest Hills: Additional doctors and nurses were dispatched to pitch in. Amato had been working day and night under tremendous stress, and on the night of March 31—her daughter's birthday—she was on the phone with Dr. John D'Angelo, the leader of emergency services for the Northwell system, explaining that at Forest Hills the scene was desperate. He responded by setting up an immediate call with all the other directors of emergency departments at all the other hospitals throughout the system. "I need you to get on the call," D'Angelo said to Dr. Amato, "and I need you to explain to everybody what's happening at your hospital."

What D'Angelo did not know was that just minutes before, Amato had been FaceTiming with one of her employees, Prea, who was critically ill at Jamaica Hospital. Jamaica Hospital, which is not part of the Northwell network, is three and a half miles away from Forest Hills. Prea, thirty-four years old, worked as a clerk in Amato's emergency department, and she had gotten very sick at home; so sick that she was about to be intubated at Jamaica Hospital. But Prea desperately wanted to be transferred to Forest Hills so that she could be cared for by her friends and coworkers. Amato's hospital was overwhelmed, but there was no way she was going to refuse a request from a member of her team. She approved the transfer, but in that moment she felt emotionally overwhelmed. "I was trying to get one of my folks back here and at the same time, I was trying to get people out," she said. "So, when John called to tell me I had to make that phone call, he didn't know that I had just been FaceTiming with my clerk in the ICU at Jamaica. And I just started crying and he said, 'can you do this?' And I said, 'I think I can. I just need a few minutes. I got this. It's just that the shit's hitting the fan here. It's crazy.'"

And it was crazy, but it would have been far crazier had D'Angelo and other leaders not already begun moving patients out of Forest Hills to other Northwell facilities a full ten days earlier. Our teams had started load balancing—moving patients from overcrowded hospitals to open beds elsewhere in our system—on Saturday, March 21, when we'd moved eight ICU patients on ventilators to other facilities. By the next day, March 22, it was clear to D'Angelo and other leaders that "we needed to offload volume from our Forest Hills and Valley Stream hospitals daily to keep them afloat." Between March 21 and 27, we transported an average of about twenty patients a day out of those hospitals. Within a few days, a total of sixty-three patients were moved out of those two hospitals to safety elsewhere.

But by March 31, inpatient capacity was still stretched beyond the limit at the Forest Hills and Valley Stream hospitals. The other hospital medical directors throughout our system had been bending over backward to help Forest Hills and Valley Stream, but now D'Angelo and his colleagues decided they had no choice but to take a radical step. If the other hospitals in our system were full and unable to take any more inpatients on their units, D'Angelo said, it was necessary to use the emergency departments at those hospitals as a "release valve for inpatients from Forest Hills." It was unusual to transfer from one hospital's inpatient units, including ICUs, to another hospital's emergency department, but it had to be done. D'Angelo wanted the other hospital emergency department leaders to hear directly from Amato how truly desperate the situation was at Forest Hills. She got on the call and reported in detail, trying to convey the harrowing nature of what was going on. After she gave them the grim picture, D'Angelo said to the doctors at the other hospitals that there was no choice but to send them each patients.

This was so unusual, said Amato. "We were going to send vented ICU patients to their emergency departments for their ED staff to take care of until they got an ICU bed at their own site. That's really asking a lot of people. You're really, literally, telling people: 'I'm about to give you the sickest of the sickest patients, and your ERs are going to have to care for them, until your hospital can get them upstairs.'" She was concerned while she was on the call that there might be some negative reactions from her counterparts. And then, after the call ended, her phone began pinging again and again as text messages rolled in from her colleagues around the system:

Just wanted to reach out and say you are doing an incredible job. What you are facing is beyond overwhelming and it is appreciated by all of us.
Thank you thank you thank you

That night, D'Angelo ordered "a parade of ambulances [to flood] the streets of those two EDs to show the staff the cavalry has arrived, and that night we moved an additional thirty-eight patients out to our other system EDs to be managed there until those hospitals had capacity to bring them to inpatient units the next day."

At Forest Hills, Amato looked outside and saw so many ambulances that the hospital security team had to go out into the street and direct traffic. "I felt like the cavalry showed up. I have no other word for it. I felt I was in a war and you look up over the mountain and the cavalry is coming down with everything you need." For the staff members, most of who had been feeling overwhelmed, it was a huge relief to see stretchers leaving the hospital and going into ambulances that would take patients to places where they would receive excellent care. An essential capability enabling us to pull this off was the workers at our central transfer center, who could dispatch scores of ambulances in minutes.

Typically, pre-coronavirus, transfers were cumbersome and time-consuming in large part because it is a highly regulated process. Under the Emergency Medical Treatment and Labor Act, in order to transfer a patient to another hospital, the sending hospital must call the desired receiving hospital to identify a receiving physician and service who agrees to the transfer; confirm the hospital has available space for that patient; and then inform the patient and obtain their consent to be transferred. Not this night at Forest Hills. In crisis lies opportunity, and the leadership team had figured out how to strip away all the unnecessary bureaucracy and move patients very quickly to safe havens in other Northwell hospitals in Westchester and Suffolk counties, Manhattan, Staten Island, and elsewhere.

The actual process for transferring patients had many moving parts. It began with an effort to identify patients at Forest Hills and Valley Stream who would be the best match for the types of beds available at receiving sites. The Northwell central transfer center, from which the ambulances were dispatched, managed the process of sending, transporting, and receiving. The central transfer center "managed all the logistics, taking as much burden off of the Forest Hills and Valley Stream staff as possible," said D'Angelo. "We placed an emergency physician in the transfer center to review the charts and determine the safety of the transfer, taking into consideration the patient's current oxygen require-ments, vital signs, and distance of potential receiving sites. We matched patients with the right receiving location and the [central transfer center] physician took care of the medical hand-off, communicating with the receiving teams. The staff at the sending sites listed patients they thought stable enough to transfer and then informed the patients and their fami-lies that they were being moved. Unlike normal times, we weren't asking the patients for permission. We were telling them they were going and that it was the safest thing for them given the volume of patients in these hospitals."

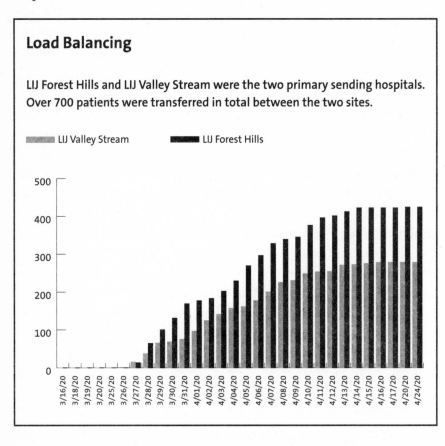

Load Balancing

LIJ Forest Hills and LIJ Valley Stream were the two primary sending hospitals. Over 700 patients were transferred in total between the two sites.

LIJ Valley Stream   LIJ Forest Hills

* * *

Throughout the crisis, there was a constant battle against fear and emo-tion among everyone on the staff. Prea, the clerk who had been transferred to Forest Hills from Jamaica Hospital, passed away several days later. She had lived with her parents and her eight-year-old twins in Queens, and at some point her mother got the virus as well. The mother of one of the Forest Hills doctors died, as did one of our nurses, a patient care assistant, and an environmental services aide.

"It was a very emotional time," Amato said. She had little time to do anything other than run her ED, but when things began to calm down toward May and she could pay attention to life beyond the hospital, she was shocked to see that questions about how to handle the disease had taken on a political dimension nationally. "When you're in it, you're just fighting it all," she said, "but when you go out into the world and you realize there's a political slant to it, I think that really, actually hurt us in the long run. I think if we had been able to be more united, it would've helped, as a country. As opposed to being divided. You think about polio and measles and where people kind of pulled together."

* * *

What would we have done at Forest Hills if the hospital had not been part of a large integrated system? Where would these patients have gone? What would have happened to them? D'Angelo said that:

> if you could think of: What is the worst-case scenario in the country? That is what happened at Forest Hills. And I think there are a lot of opportunities and lessons to be learned from Forest Hills, and I don't know what a hospital like Forest Hills does if they are in that situation and they don't have the mutual aid of all the other hospitals in our system. I literally have this vision of people dying in the streets in lines waiting to get in. I just don't know how they would have survived. I can't even imagine what the mortality rate would be in that community if it weren't for the fact that we were able to [relieve] them of a significant number of patients so that they can tread water as much as they had to.

Over a four-week period, 423 very sick patients from Forest Hills, and 278 from Valley Stream, many on ventilators, were moved to alternative hospitals.

Why were we able to handle the onslaught when, twenty minutes away, at Elmhurst Hospital, they were overwhelmed? There were many reasons. Public hospitals in the city had been underfunded for years and thus lacked the resources we had for emergency management. But a key element was also preparation and the training that goes with it. Said Susan Browning:

> I think, internally, we had done so much advanced planning for emergencies, and we had done so much training within the four walls, that we kind of clicked into how to respond. Beyond our four walls, there's no way we could have handled this if we had not had the ability to transfer patients within our health system. So, the fact that we are a member of an integrated health system and were able to transfer patients out seamlessly, is what allowed us to be able to function at the level that we were functioning locally.

Said Northwell Vice President and Chief Administrative Officer Gene Tangney: "All the training we did gave us muscle memory."

* * *

A terrible price was paid for the work we did during the crisis. And we may not yet be done paying it. Amid the extreme sickness and the deaths of patients, there was always fear. At the start, the staff did not know what to expect. They were well aware that many patients in Italy and China had died, and they were also acutely aware that many health-care workers just like themselves had succumbed to the virus. But it was nevertheless devastating to have our colleagues at Forest Hills get infected and lose their lives. Joyce, a labor and delivery nurse manager, tested positive, as did her adult sons and her husband. At home, her condition deteriorated to the point where her husband had to dress her to bring her to the hospital. The emergency department team was on alert for her arrival. When she arrived, she was in cardiogenic shock. She was intubated, went into full cardiac arrest, and died.

At Forest Hills, a pregnant woman near full term was in extreme respiratory distress. The OB team gave her a spinal and did an emergency C-section and brought a healthy baby into the world. The mother was then intubated and survived. There was one case, however, where a pregnant mother delivered her child and then succumbed to the disease. Her husband passed away as well. In normal times, that would have been such a tragic story that our teams would have been talking about it and little else for a month. But in the crisis it was just another story. Those on the front lines of the crisis will likely be reckoning with the impact of their experiences, and of the many heartbreaking losses, for a long time to come.

CHAPTER TWO

A Culture of Preparedness

Lessons
- Establishing an emergency operations center (EOC) and Incident Command System (ICS) similar to that used by the military and managed by experienced professionals is imperative.
- Emergency preparedness must be ingrained as a core part of the culture and competence of the organization. It cannot be put in place effectively during a crisis.
- A daily dashboard with key data and metrics is essential to successful operations. (See Daily Dashboard Metrics in Appendix II.)
- In a crisis, throw the budget out the window. Deal with it later.
- Train and prepare until your organization is "comfortable with being uncomfortable."
- Marshal essential resources including people, supplies, and financial resilience to sustain a lengthy siege. Prepare and act early.

In the years since we built our emergency system, we have been tested numerous times. On September 11, 2001, we were ready within hours of the attacks, expecting (incorrectly) that we would be inundated with casualties. In August of 2003 the power grid in the northeastern part of the United States failed, the nation's worst blackout ever. We went into incident command mode and every backup generator at Northwell facilities kicked in on cue, with a single exception. And because we had a backup plan to our backup plan, we had another generator to bring online in lieu of the one that failed. (Part of the preparation had also included agreements with a variety of vendors—including fuel suppliers—that fuel would remain available under any and all circumstances.) In late October 2012, Superstorm Sandy barreled up the East Coast, leaving widespread devastation in its wake. When two of our hospitals were threatened with flooding, we were able to evacuate hundreds of patients, many from ICUs, and transport them to other hospitals within our system where they were safe. Other hospitals outside of our system were overwhelmed by the storm, and we helped move some of their patients to safety, as well.

We also activated our emergency response teams when the country was threatened with Ebola, H1N1, and severe acute respiratory syndrome (SARS). In response to the Ebola threat, we built an isolation unit and designed PPE featured on the front page of the *New York Times* and promoted in Congress. When the SARS virus appeared in 2003, hitting Canada particularly hard, we sent one of our leaders to Toronto to learn. Mary Mahoney, vice president of emergency management, found that some of the health-care workers who were dying were actually infecting themselves because of the flawed method they used in donning and doffing PPE. "So that was a lesson we brought back to the health system," Mahoney said, "and we started a big push on donning and doffing PPE properly. We also built hospital surge plans, asking: Where else could we put patients in an emergency? What types of equipment would we need, and supplies? And we started building a small cache of that."

In short, we have thought about, discussed, and planned for a virus arriving in New York from Asia so often that a 2017 book about some of our work noted:

> At Northwell there is a particular sensitivity to monitoring the existence and scope of infectious diseases no matter where in the world they might exist. Northwell's proximity to three large international airports—JFK, LaGuardia, Newark—place major points of entry to the U.S. within minutes of Northwell

hospitals. A passenger arriving from Asia with bird flu, or one travelling from Africa with symptoms of Ebola, could well arrive on the Northwell doorstep.

When our surveillance team saw the development of a new virus in Wuhan, China, in January 2020, we began pulling our emergency operation together. Many people think of China as the other side of the world, seven thousand miles from New York, but in our command center we think of it as a half-day plane ride. As we monitored from a distance, we pulled out the manual from our SARS experience that we had shared with the state and began to update contingency plans. We checked inventories and purchased additional supplies of PPE, ventilators, and other material. We acted absolutely as if it was happening, with complete dedication to getting as ready as we could get.

That said, did we ever think we would have to build thousands of new beds, transport hundreds of patients out of jam-packed hospitals, and fight in a bare-knuckle marketplace against other hospital systems and states and the federal government for equipment? Or that we would have to shut down virtually our entire system to care for COVID patients? Or see people dying without their loved ones allowed to visit in their final moments? Or that fifty-cent masks would cost seven dollars? Or that we would have staff members die from the disease they were treating?

Never in our wildest imagination did we envision a force so malevolent.

We possessed a number of assets that gave us confidence in our preparations: an experienced emergency management team; a reliable structure in which the team operated; a twenty-three-hospital network; and large supplies of equipment and PPE. We also felt prepared psychologically because we are an organization that is, in the words of Chief of Administration Gene Tangney, "comfortable with being uncomfortable" in an emergency. We were guided by real-time data that our emergency team reviewed at the beginning and end of each day. Our main dashboard gave us all of the information our team needed to make rapid decisions.

We were guided by the mantra of Northwell Chief Operating Officer Mark Solazzo: "Our priorities from the start were, number one, keep the staff safe and informed; number two, keep our facilities safe; and number three, be able to take care of anyone who comes to us needing care." But this was catastrophic history in real time: a pandemic for which we had no prevention or treatment; and a virus whose means of transmission was initially a mystery, powerful enough to destroy the lungs of even the healthiest among us. At the start we knew next to nothing about the disease. We did not yet know how devastating it could be, nor that it could damage the liver or clot the blood. We did not fully understand the impact of a sustained, round-the-clock assault on our inpatient hospital units, on our emergency departments, and on our eight hundred ambulatory sites. The last time something like this had struck—the so-called Spanish flu, 103 years before—fifty million people worldwide had been struck down.

From the start, we knew that the virus was moving quickly and we knew that we could not allow it to get ahead of us. We raced against this virus as it sprinted around the globe, headed directly for our communities. We had to run fast enough to stay ahead of it, if only by a half-step, and thus our emergency team set off on a sprint that was destined to last for months. As any athlete knows, sprinting all out for a hundred yards or so is doable. Sprinting all out for miles and miles, which is what this experience was like, is something else altogether. Every time we thought we were putting distance between ourselves and the wave, the virus would crest right there, seemingly just inches behind us as we ran to stay ahead—supplying PPE to keep our staff safe, creating new beds for patients, finding ventilators to keep people alive, and reassigning staff. The right attitude helped. Confidence and optimism are products of rigorous preparation and, though humbled, we remained confident throughout.

"Systemness" was essential to our identity, and that integration allowed us to consolidate functions, standardize best practices, and move team members and equipment wherever needed, as we saw in chapter 1. Even with all of this in addition to a culture of emergency preparedness, we were still stretched to our limits by the crisis. But we were guided throughout by the steadiness and reliability of our incident command structure—the foundation of our emergency response capability.

The Northwell Emergency Operations Center Incident Management System is led by the incident commander, Northwell COO Mark

Solazzo, and Deputy Incident Commander Gene Tangney. Both have extensive emergency preparedness experience; in fact, both started their careers as emergency medical technicians. The incident command structure is virtually identical to the structure used by police and fire departments, by FEMA, and by many military organizations. It makes lines of command and responsibilities clear and is essential to our ability to make the well-informed, rapid decisions that are key to successful emergency management.

The command structure is organized simply:

- Operations include hospital, clinical, and ambulatory services and post-acute services; post-acute services include home care after hospitalization.
- Finance and Administration include legal affairs and costs and expenses.
- Planning includes human resources, staffing, employee health services, and team member contact tracing and data.
- Logistics includes procurement, facilities, and communications.

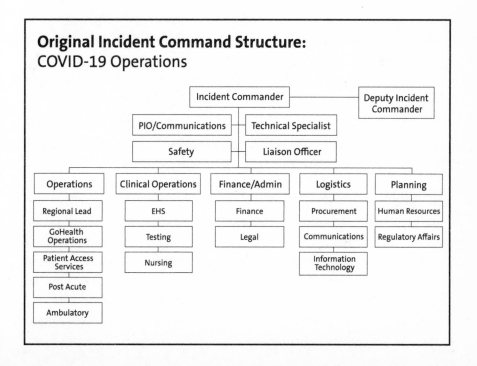

Original Incident Command Structure:
COVID-19 Operations

One of the reasons this approach works is because every one of these functional areas is represented on the emergency committee. And everyone in the group understands that when the team is called up, the normal rules of business are suspended and we work in a more streamlined, urgent manner. This may appear less collaborative than our traditional approach, but there is much collaboration within the committee—very rapid collaboration—and then the incident commander issues an order and we proceed. The process removes any form of bureaucracy, which enables the team to work faster and more efficiently.

Part of our emergency preparedness includes a monitoring and early-warning capability. We watched events in Wuhan closely, and when it was clear the threat was growing, we sounded the alarm even before the state government did, convening our team on January 21 in our emergency operations center in Great Neck, Long Island. This space, with its extensive communications network, is the location from which the team managed previous emergencies, working shoulder to shoulder in one room with experts from every area of the health system.

Then, suddenly and quite unexpectedly, our emergency operations command structure was disrupted. Weeks before the first confirmed cases, the virus stealthily arrived from Europe and penetrated the New York area in mid-February. We were about to separate our senior leadership team to ensure continuity of operations when the

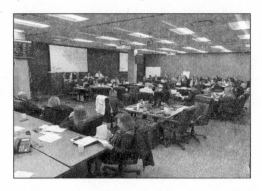

Pictured is our original emergency operations center in Great Neck, Long Island.

virus beat us to the punch: Two members of our leadership team got sick and tested positive for the virus. This required many members of the team to quarantine. At this point we had little understanding about the nature of the virus and the disease it caused. We didn't yet understand its virulence or speed or means of transmission, and we certainly were not aware of any effective treatment. This lack of knowledge made many of the team members extremely uncomfortable. It was a jarring moment that humbled a seasoned group confident in its abilities. We were now prevented from meeting in person where we had worked well and comfortably together. We were forced, overnight, to shift into a virtual world. This was a real blow, for it meant not only that key members of our team, including our Incident Commander Mark Solazzo, had to isolate from office and family; it also meant we had to get up to speed on meeting effectively in cyberspace. Gene Tangney, the deputy incident commander, believed that a team mentality and an inclusive leadership culture were the foundation of our health system success. When in the past the team was together in the command center, there was something powerful about the closeness and camaraderie of the members being physically together, making decisions under stress face-to-face. Now that key component was lost.

"This virus challenged one of the core foundational strengths of our health system: the ability to act as a team physically together managing whatever challenge we were given," Tangney said. "Once we learned that several key members of our leadership group were compromised by the virus we were thrust into this new environment. This was extremely challenging at first. I equate it to writing with your nondominant hand—it just didn't feel comfortable."

With no more in-person meetings, the team now had to adapt to virtual gatherings via Microsoft Teams, a program with which most of the men and women on our team were unfamiliar. The initial sessions were awkward. But the IT team connected every member of our group and offered guidance, and we adapted. It was especially helpful that the application enabled team members to see and hear one another as well as to share documents online.

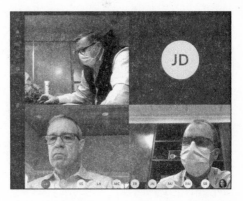

The leadership team quickly transitioned to virtual meetings through Microsoft Teams.

* * *

It was unsettling to get knocked off stride right at the start. But the team quickly adapted to the new reality and managed effectively. This was, after all, a viral threat, and for twenty years we had placed such threats at or near the top of anticipated disasters for which the team had prepared. New York is the crossroads of the world. There are international travelers twenty minutes from our hospitals, housing density unlike anywhere else in the United States, jam-packed subways, streets, restaurants, and theaters. It's as though New York was designed as the ideal virus transmission vehicle. It turned out that four members of the emergency management team were infected; fortunately, all recovered and returned to work.

Senior people in our organization had warned us about this type of virus and worse. Dr. Kevin Tracey, a neurosurgeon who heads our Feinstein Institutes for Medical Research at Northwell and who was intimately involved in all aspects of responding to the crisis, possessed a fascinating perspective based on his experiences during the SARS crisis. SARS (severe acute respiratory syndrome) first appeared in southern China in November 2002, spreading to twenty-six countries and infecting 8,098 people within months. The disease, which manifested in pneumonia or respiratory distress syndrome, was caused by a then-new coronavirus. It had a high mortality rate (nearly 10 percent) but a low rate of infection. A few months after SARS was first identified, in early 2003, Tracey was invited to a confidential meeting of a select number of senior scientists at the Defense Advanced Research Projects Agency (DARPA), a division of the United States Department of Defense headquartered in Arlington, Virginia. Included in the meeting were Drs. Michael Callahan and Robert Kadlec, both of whom, along with Tracey, would play important roles in the coronavirus drama of 2020. The physicians were asked by the DARPA officials: "How should the federal government prepare for a virus with high mortality rates (10 percent or greater) and *high* infectivity?"

After some deliberation that day and some calculations on a whiteboard, "we recommended establishing stockpiles of one to two million ventilators, PPE, and stockpiles of broad spectrum antibiotics and intravenous saline sufficient for ten to twenty million people," Tracey said. In the event of a rapidly spreading, highly lethal, airborne virus, potentially arriving in only one person on an incoming flight, the effect of a new virus would be the deaths of a significant portion of the population (25–40 percent) within six months. If unchecked, supply chains would fail, doctors and nurses would die and not be available to treat the sick, and hospitals would be overrun and fail. In that scenario, the only option would be to put the sick in local schools, fire stations, or tents, deploy the supplies from the stockpile, and hope that sufficient human expertise would be available to utilize the resources locally. "We told them to buy millions of jetpack ventilators like the Green Berets carry and put them in stockpiles strategically distributed around the United States," Tracey recalled. If all of those recommendations had been put into place, perhaps the country might have been better prepared.

* * *

By February 2020, the news out of Italy was unsettling. Projections for our area were concerning, and then alarming. We accelerated our preparation and took a series of steps in anticipation of the virus's arrival, and we did so well before we were mandated by government to do anything. We:

- threw our organizational budget out the window and vowed to spend whatever it took to get the supplies and people we needed;
- spent millions on additional PPE for our staff;
- connected very early in the crisis with staffing companies and signed contracts to hire hundreds of additional nurses from around the country for the months ahead;
- booked hundreds of hotel rooms to accommodate these nurses and other staff members who wanted to avoid going home where they could infect family members;
- upped our surge plan to create bed capacity far beyond our normal ability;
- canceled all travel for Northwell staff and pulled team members back from medical missions around the globe;
- began working in our laboratory to develop a test to determine which patients were COVID-19 positive;
- discharged any patients who could safely recuperate at home;

- canceled all elective surgeries—tens of thousands of planned operations of people seeking new knees, hips, and much more. In fact, we canceled elective surgeries before it was mandated by the state. We did it for safety reasons, of course, but we also did it in anticipation of needing to redeploy the bedside staff.
- communicated with all staff members exactly what we saw coming and how we were preparing.

The result of these moves, in just a matter of days, was that our hospitals had fewer non-COVID patients than ever before—two thousand empty beds in a system where we typically run at, and sometimes just over, 100 percent capacity. On the eve of the outbreak, our hallways were quiet, many rooms empty.

Michelle Cusack, our chief financial officer, recalled that "back in February, we thought the disruption might be in the tens of millions of dollars, but within three or four short days that went from tens of millions to hundreds of millions in terms of disruption, in terms of dollars gone, revenue gone." In consultation with other senior leaders, Cusack made the decision to immediately draw down on our lines of credit to increase our liquidity and at the same time to increase our lines up to eight hundred million dollars. In fact, noted Mark Solazzo, total revenue loss and increased expenses—in just a three-month period—totaled $1.6 billion.

Preparation goes a long way in an emergency, but this threat was different from anything we—or anyone else—had experienced. Most emergencies happen quickly and are short-lived. A flood inundates the area and then it recedes, and full recovery efforts are underway in forty-eight hours. And with a flood the disaster is confined to one part of the country. Thus, emergency supplies and personnel can move in from elsewhere and help out the impacted locale. The coronavirus was obviously very different: It hit hard, but then harder still as time passed, and not for hours or days but for weeks, then months. And it struck the entire world, forcing organizations globally to compete against one another for people and supplies. In floods and similar disasters, hospitals are rarely tested beyond their capacity, but this was different, and as February turned to March it seemed more than likely that the virus would make many

New Yorkers sick. In fact, the projections absent social distancing and other mitigation were for numbers of sick patients that would have overwhelmed the region's health-care system.

As we prepared, there was a lamentable if predictable moment—one that seems to happen during the preparation period for every emergency—when, during the relative calm before the storm, some people suffer from unhelpful skepticism. As much as we are confident in our culture of preparedness, there are always a few dissenting voices who question whether we are overreacting. *Will the hurricane coming up the coast turn out to sea and miss us entirely? Will the Ebola virus get here or not? Do we really need to disrupt the entire enterprise for something that may not even get here?* In other words: *Is all this really necessary?*

The answer came from reports out of Italy, cruise ships, and events in Seattle where patients at a nursing home were struck down. Now instead of skeptical questions, people asked: *How many flights from Italy and Seattle into JFK every day?* And then it was clear that projections from various sources—the state government, private consultancies, academics, and our own analysis—indicated that this could be a perfect storm. In light of the contagious nature of the virus and, at the time, out of an abundance of caution, we directed thirty thousand of our seventy-two thousand employees to work from home, including personnel from office-based operations such as billing, legal, IT, and others.

On March 4, with the tidal wave about to strike, we set up a twenty-four/seven call center focused entirely on coronavirus-related questions and concerns. Panic was building among the public, and we were inundated with calls. People needed answers and we were able to set up and train call center staff with detailed information on the virus within forty-eight hours. This proved to be an important asset throughout the crisis, because it allowed our patients to access us quickly and get the answers they needed. *Should I cancel a doctor's appointment? What are the criteria for getting tested?* The call center had barely started when its volume escalated to 4,500 calls a day, says Dr. John D'Angelo, "with nurses doing risk assessment on the patients that were calling in and referring those that required evaluation to our urgent care network, which was a plan to try to protect the hospitals from their EDs being overwhelmed." We typically answered calls within thirty seconds and most callers were

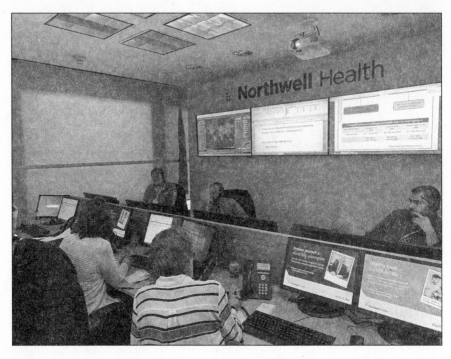

Pictured is our 24/7 COVID call center with staff actively talking to patients.

satisfied with our help. Some callers were quite upset that tests were unavailable, but that was due to the federal government having stumbled out of the gate with a faulty test. Some callers with technical medical questions were referred to nurses. And the call center proved to be even more valuable when testing started to become more widely available. Call center nurses, upon receiving test results on a particular patient electronically, would call that patient and inform them what the result was and what they should do; for example, remain home for a period of time. At one point, with call volume growing rapidly, the call center leaders asked for seventy to eighty additional nurses to be assigned to the phones. At Northwell, we have an internal staffing company called Flexstaff that keeps track of employees available for additional shifts or even new assignments. Early on, we were able to fill the need for nurses at the call center through Flexstaff, but it was soon clear that critical care and emergency medicine nurses were urgently needed at the front lines. We turned to forty newly minted nurses just out of our graduate school of nursing and physician assistant studies that we operate jointly with

Hofstra University, and the young nurses handled the phone assignments with great skill.

* * *

In early March, the virus struck Greater New York. A lawyer in New Rochelle, a suburban community not far from New York City, fell ill, and soon the governor took unprecedented action to lock down the New Rochelle community, which had quickly become a viral hot spot. At the governor's request, our Northwell team in partnership with the state set up a drive-through testing center for people within the town to determine whether they, too, had been infected.

Just three days later, on Friday, March 6, Dr. John D'Angelo was scheduled for an interview in Manhattan with the ABC News program *20/20*. He arrived that night at the Northwell freestanding emergency department in Greenwich Village where he planned to spend some time with the staff and see how things were going. The charge nurse approached him and told him that there was a possibility they had just gotten their first case of the virus. The patient presented with severe respiratory distress, but he did not have any of the other indications which, according to CDC guidelines at the time, would make him a likely candidate for testing. That is, he had not traveled internationally, had not had known contact with a person who had the virus, and did not have a fever.

The CDC testing guidelines also contained a kind of "catch-all category" which said that patients should be tested "if in a doctor's judgement there was a possibility they were positive." This was an exceedingly vague standard, and D'Angelo had already been concerned about it. What if there were COVID-positive patients who checked none of the CDC boxes, arrived in the ED, and were later determined to have the virus? That type of patient would infect receptionists and nurses and doctors in the ED—anyone with whom he had interacted. In other words, D'Angelo realized, patients *who did not fit the profile* could well shed virus throughout an entire emergency department, sickening critical health-care workers.

That night, when the charge nurse said she thought they might have their first patient, D'Angelo was watching the staff "walk the patient from a regular room—not an isolation room—down the hall and put him in an isolation room, and as they're telling me the story, the patient had already been there for two hours." The patient had a history of asthma and had thought it was just his normal asthma acting up. The team was treating him, but he kept wheezing, and, despite usual treatment, was worsening as time went on. The treating physician ordered a CT scan of his chest, thinking maybe he was suffering from something other than his usual asthma, and the scan revealed the ground-glass appearance said to be common with COVID-19-positive patients. This patient, a man in his fifties who believed he was suffering from asthma, deteriorated so rapidly as the virus attacked his lungs that he had to be placed on a ventilator the next day.

It was determined that six staff members in the ED had been exposed to the patient and were sent home to isolate. Several of the staff subsequently got sick, though luckily none seriously. That night it became clear to D'Angelo that any patient walking into any of our emergency departments—whether they had traveled anywhere or not, whether they checked the

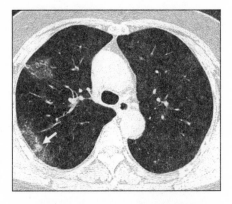

Normal Lungs, Source: *Business Insider*

symptom boxes from the CDC or not—might be a carrier of the virus. This was, to say the least, alarming, for it meant that literally any person walking in the door of any of our emergency departments might be a threat to our staff. And if that were the case, D'Angelo realized, then every staff person and every patient in all of our EDs had to be masked to prevent the

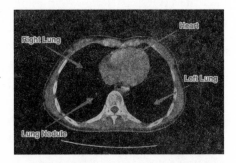

CT X-ray of lungs infected with COVID-19, Source: *Business Insider*

spread. N95 masks were preferred, but even a procedural mask would, in D'Angelo's words, give the staff a fighting chance: "They're not going to know these patients are positive until two hours later," he said, "because it's impossible to know the end result until you do the work-up and the patient progresses."

The smart choice was to behave as though every patient who walked through the door had the virus, and, on that presumption, D'Angelo wanted every employee in every Northwell ED to start wearing a mask at all times. The policy was issued the following day:

> The rationale for just instituting the policy in the emergency department was that, in the emergency department, we see people that are undifferentiated; they just show up at the door and say, 'I'm here for X,' and then it takes time to work them up to figure out what they really have. Whereas people admitted to the hospital have had a work-up, X-rays, other testing, and we already know they have pneumonia, or something else.

Up to that point, the number of emergency department team members out sick and suspected of having the virus had been steadily climbing. After the mask mandate was put in place, many fewer staff members got sick, even as the number of patients increased at a staggering rate in the weeks ahead.

Surprisingly, our mask mandate actually caused something of a rift with the other health systems worried about their supply. If we were using many more masks than usual, which we were, could they end up shorthanded? At other systems, there was a concern that employees might say *they're wearing masks at Northwell, why aren't we?* One of the other major health systems in New York actually put out a video to their staff on the proper use of PPE and noted in it, as D'Angelo remembered it, "something like: 'some organizations in our region are doing things that aren't rational and aren't based on science,' the implication being that what we were doing was irresponsible." But about a week later the CDC came out with a new guideline that having patients and staff in masks would make an exposure to an unknown COVID patient go from a high-risk to a low-risk exposure. D'Angelo's decision was a game changer. It was one of those lessons that we learned and put into practice immediately that wound up keeping our staff much safer than they would have been otherwise. In retrospect, it is clear that the masking order protected many employees and patients.

* * *

Before the virus struck New York, our health system functioned efficiently on many different levels. Our doctors in every conceivable specialty treated patients. Surgeons operated. Mental health professionals cared for patients in psychiatric units. In other words, seventy-two thousand people went about the business of caring for tens of thousands of patients with hundreds and hundreds of different medical conditions. And then, virtually overnight, everything changed. We went from normalcy to battle stations; to converting virtually our entire system into the country's largest COVID-focused health system, where our emergency departments, medical surgical beds, and ICU beds were all packed with COVID-19 patients. Our hospitals had become COVID hospitals. Had we ever experienced anything quite like this? Had anyone?

Dr. Mark Jarrett, Northwell chief quality officer, had a reaction to the onslaught that was shared by many physicians within our system: "As it ramped up we knew it was getting worse, but in forty-two years of professional life, I have never had to address anything that is so much illness and potential death. It's just unbelievable. It really, literally, is the hardest thing we have ever had to do."

Gene Tangney has spent his professional life in emergency services, and after he had a chance in early May to reflect upon the crisis, he acknowledged how harrowing it had been. But he also identified some things that worked well for us. He wrote in a memo after the virus had passed the peak:

> If this pandemic has taught us one thing it's that organizations that have a strong emergency preparedness structure and culture fared better than organizations that just checked the boxes and didn't truly accept the foundational elements of preparedness into their operations. Emergency response requires flexibility, commitment, and an innovative culture to truly successfully manage large scale disasters. This culture needs to

start from the top of the organization. . . . Our health system leaders have championed the culture of emergency preparedness. . . . Having seasoned leaders that are empowered and are willing to make decisions in the toughest times can be the difference between successfully or unsuccessfully managing an event.

CHAPTER THREE

An Integrated System

Lessons

- Scale is important, but more important is the ability within an integrated system to be able to use the scale to full advantage. Organizations need to develop an integrated sense of *"systemness."*
- With an integrated system, you have the ability to *load balance*— that is, move patients where they are safest and will get the best care.
- With an integrated system you have the ability to deploy your most important resources—staff and equipment—where most needed.
- Build an ambulance system with trained staff capable of transporting ICU patients from one facility to another over various distances. An ambulance system is an integrator, knitting together the whole system.
- Nurses, physicians, and other staff on the front lines are capable of learning entirely new competencies and management skills in the midst of crisis.
- This integrated team approach has to be fostered over time; it cannot be initiated in the midst of a crisis.

When the tsunami struck we were able to cope thanks to the scale and integration of our health system. Dr. Ira Nash, executive director of Northwell Physician Partners, put it this way:

> Scale is necessary, but it is hardly sufficient. What I believe distinguished the Northwell effort is the *utilization* of scale, which was possible only because of our true integration . . . coupled with a sense of obligation to support all parts of the organization. I have heard stories of other health "systems" (which also have scale) but which failed to execute the way we did because they either lacked true integration (unified leadership) and/or, when push came to shove, some parts of the organization were valued more than others.

As Nash pointed out, the integrated nature of our organization enabled us to load balance; that is, to distribute patients to anywhere within our system where beds were available.

At the very early stages of the crisis, Governor Cuomo was pushing all health systems in the state to increase capacity by a minimum of 50 percent. He asked one of us (Michael Dowling) to team up with Ken Raske, head of the Greater New York Hospital Association, and to work with hospitals throughout the state to achieve that goal. The governor joined calls with the heads of every hospital in New York to urge action. In addition to that group, the governor asked us to coordinate actions with the major New York City systems including Mount Sinai, New York Presbyterian, NYU, Montefiore, and Northwell. The leaders of these organizations would gather to confer on a conference call three times a week.

The governor's bed surge goal was aggressive, but we and most other systems were eventually able to meet it. Just how aggressive a target was it? Mark Solazzo asked his team of analysts in late March to update their data and predict how many additional beds we would need at the apex. The answer came back: You need to create at least two hundred new beds every day for the next eight days. In other words, push our total beds from 3,100 up toward the 5,000-bed range. To comply with the governor's request we transformed conference rooms, recovery rooms, and waiting areas into clinical treatment sites. The bed expansion at North Shore University Hospital, the largest in our system, reflected the urgent nature of the task at hand. "We just started to claim units with no negotiation with any services in the building," said Jon Sendach, head of North Shore. "This is a major academic medical center, which typically does not run as an autocratic type of a setup." It was, to say the least, atypical for Sendach and the chief medical officer, Dr. Michael Gitman, to be issuing orders absent much consultation. In fact, it was exactly contrary to the collaborative culture Sendach and Gitman had worked to build. But there was no choice. "We had to just very quickly start to do things. When you're in a situation where you need beds now for incoming ER arrivals, it becomes very, very, important that you have individuals who say, 'I understand.' And we had that here throughout."

People pitched in from departments across the North Shore campus. Part of North Shore includes Katz Women's Hospital, a dedicated obstetrics (OB) facility. As the crisis was approaching, "our OB leadership said, 'Hey, wait a second. We'll get out of the way. We have all these beds and private rooms for our antepartum and postpartum patients,' and we hatched this plan to move all the OB patients to an ambulatory surgery

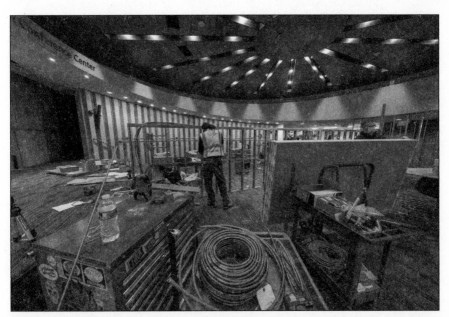

Pictured is the Rust Auditorium being actively dismantled and constructed into a patient unit.

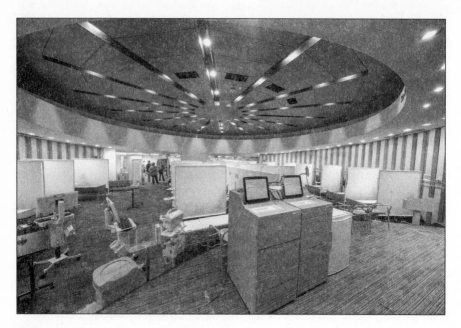

Many makeshift overflow units like the one pictured here at Rust Auditorium existed throughout the system.

center in another building on our campus." This would make room for COVID patients and, at the same time, keep mothers and babies away from the virus. Sendach also directed that the auditorium within the hospital be dismantled and turned into patient treatment areas. Rows of seats, 250 in all, were bolted to the floor and needed to be unbolted, moved, and stored. Then we needed to turn the space into a clinical area for sick patients. North Shore University Hospital is such a large institution that included within its staff is an engineering group, including engineers, carpenters, electricians, and plumbers who are capable of amazing work. The team assessed the situation, consulted, drew up a plan, and got to work. They unbolted and removed every seat, constructed a series of walls, ran electric power into the patient cubicles, and installed privacy screens between beds—screens that were built overnight in the workshop using PVC pipe and plastic drapes. Sendach had the team take the sofa beds that fathers slept on at the women's hospital, had them cleaned, and installed them in the auditorium. Incredibly, the team completed the entire reconstruction project in under twenty-four hours.

The surge of patients throughout our system was so great that during the third week in March we had about one hundred COVID patients in all our hospitals; two weeks later we had nearly three thousand and we had yet to reach the peak. The *New York Times* reported at the time: "Across the city, hospitals are overrun. Patients have died in hallways before they could even be hooked up to one of the few available ventilators in New York. Doctors and nurses, who have had to use the same protective gear again and again, are getting sick. So many people are dying that the city is running low on body bags."[*] No longer was anyone in our system asking if all the disruption involved in preparing for an emergency was worth the trouble.

* * *

The Forest Hills example described in chapter 1 typifies what happened throughout our system. When smaller hospitals such as Forest Hills and Valley Stream were pushed to the brink, patients were transferred to some of our other hospitals in Staten Island, Westchester, and elsewhere via our transport system, which saved lives—perhaps many lives.

This movement of patients to safer locations was possible due to the integrated nature of our system. What does that mean exactly? At a basic level, all of our administrative support structures across the health system are governed centrally including administration, clinical, purchasing, legal, IT, and HR. This saves money and is more efficient than each of our twenty-three hospitals going out on their own to purchase equipment and supplies, IT systems, etc. More significantly, integration means that we establish system-wide policies for all major areas—human resources, clinical policies and guidelines, budgeting and finance, legal affairs, and more. But the secret sauce of integration is a culture of willingness among all of the various parts of the organization to support and cooperate with one another. This stands in sharp contrast to the typically siloed nature of many modern health-care entities. Our systemness gives us the ability to do things such as load balance without having to seek broad consensus or fight through bureaucratic pushback. We have few turf battles at

---

[*] Michael Rothfeld, Somini Sengupta, Joseph Goldstein, and Brian M. Rosenthal "An 'Apocalyptic' Surge at a New York Hospital," *New York Times*, March 26, 2020, updated April 14, 2020.

Northwell because no one department owns any of the turf; we all own all of the turf and that is a very rare thing indeed in health care.

The other key element of systemness is that we have within our organization the capability to care for any type of patient at any time depending upon that patient's condition and needs. For example, we can care for very sick patients in our ICUs while at the other end of the spectrum, we provide follow-up home care to patients who have been released from the hospital. We provide psychiatric care in our mental health hospitals, and we provide nursing home and hospice care to patients needing those levels of service. Because all of these capabilities are within our system, we never have to rely on others outside to care for our patients. We share not only beds and staff but also knowledge and experience.

The load-balancing process that we began to implement that terrible night in Forest Hills was modified further on the go, and the modification proved effective. "In the process we learned how to do it more quickly," said Mark Solazzo. "A normal transfer takes maybe six hours. You call for the ambulance, call for the doctor at the other site, the sending doctor gives a report to the doctor at the receiving hospital, the nurse gives a report to the receiving nurse, they package the patient and move the patient to the unit. We shortcut all of that after the first three or four days" to make the process work much faster. We always knew in real-time what the numbers were in our facilities based on our information system: how many people were waiting in any of our emergency departments, wait times, number of admissions, available beds, and COVID-positive patients. Each morning and afternoon the command group reviewed the data and moved patients from crowded or overcrowded facilities to open beds elsewhere. At the peak of the crisis, we succeeded in moving an estimated 780 patients out of the hardest-hit community hospitals to other parts of our system.

"It became the only way that our system would be able to survive," said Steve Bello, regional executive director of Northwell's eastern region. Each morning, Bello would get on the phone with Dr. John D'Angelo as well as with the leaders of the other two regions—Kevin Beiner, regional executive director in the west, and Dr. Jason Naidich, regional executive director in the central region—and they would look at fresh data generated by all of the hospitals. The data dashboard told

Load Balancing Sending and Reveiving

March 21st – April 22nd

Sending Hospital (group)	#
Glen Cove Hospital	7
Huntington Hospital	4
Lenox Hill Hospital	19
Long Island Jewish Forest Hills	423
Long Island Jewish Valley Stream	278
Long Island Jewish Medical Center	7
North Shore University Hospital	5
Southside Hospital	37
Syosset Hospital	30

810 Patients Transferred

Receiving Hospital (group)	#
Glen Cove Hospital	21
Huntington Hospital	80
Lenox Hill Hospital	169
Lenox Health Greenwich Village	25
Lenox Hill Hospital	2
Long Island Jewish	40
Long Island Jewish Medical Center	2
Mather Hospital	90
Northern Westchester Hospital	69
North Shore University Hospital	96
Peconic Bay Medical Center	92
Phelps Hospital	37
Plainview Hospital	9
Staten Island University Hospital- North & South	40
Southside Hospital	30
Syosset Hospital	8

them exactly how many patients needed to be moved and where there were openings to send them. "When we were really at the peak of load balancing, we'd move about fifty patients a day out of both Forest

Hills and Valley Stream," said Bello. "I pulled my team together out east and I said, 'We're going to be accepting patients from our sister hospitals. Be ready.' And that was it."

One problem that arose, said Bello, was how best to get recovered patients back from distant hospitals. For example, how does a patient who had been sent from Forest Hills hospital to our Peconic Bay Medical Center in Riverhead on the eastern end of Long Island near the Hamptons get back home? This was more than sixty miles from Forest Hills and, depending upon where the patient lived, could be eight or ninety miles from their residence. "Talk about culture shock," said Bello. "One day you walk into the emergency room at Forest Hills Hospital, two weeks later, you wake up in a foreign country, in Riverhead." All patients from distant hospitals were returned to their homes via ambulance.

Beds were only one part of the equation. We needed the right staff at the receiving end of the trip to be able to care for the incoming patient. This complex assignment fell to Maureen White, executive vice president and chief nurse executive, and Joe Moscola, head of HR. Once the regional leaders and Emergency Services Director John D'Angelo decided which patients were going where, it was then up to White and Moscola to make sure the beds were properly staffed. Sometimes they drew from our internal teams from idle surgical or ambulatory units. Other times they relied upon national staffing companies and contracted for several hundred nurses from around the country on short-term contracts. We

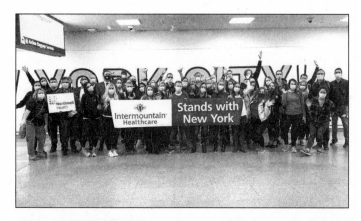

Pictured here is the Intermountain team arriving in New York to aid in the fight with Northwell Health.

graduated the class from our medical school—the Donald and Barbara Zucker School of Medicine at Hofstra/Northwell—early, and the newly minted young physicians went right to work. As a result of relationships developed by our staff members with officials from other health systems, we were fortunate to have teams from the University of Rochester and Intermountain Healthcare in Utah come to our aid, as well.

D'Angelo put the load-balancing initiative in a broader perspective. "We moved the equivalent of a tertiary level hospital," he said, "780 beds of inpatients, out of that epicenter through our central transfer process. Otherwise I don't know what would have happened. They would have been shut down; they just couldn't have handled the volume they would have been managing. And even with all that, they were stretched to capacity. I think that was a huge success of the operation."

It is important to note that our work to distribute patients and assist other hospitals went beyond our own system. Steve Bello, for example, was asked to help out our neighbor, Jamaica Hospital in Queens, one of the areas hardest hit by the coronavirus. "They were trying to get several dozen patients out of Jamaica Hospital primarily because their oxygen farm could not keep up with demand and people were at risk, and there was really nobody else that they could turn to for help. So things broadened out from within our health system to now, 'Hey, we're going to help load-balance across our region.' And that really became something significant. We helped them throughout the whole process." We were able to help them get patients into the Javits Center in Manhattan, the massive convention center that was turned into a thousand-bed field hospital in order to relieve pressure on New York's hospitals. Additional relief came when the federal government dispatched the USNS *Comfort*, a Navy hospital ship, to New York Harbor. "We embedded somebody from the Javits Center into [Jamaica Hospital]to help them along, we sent our facilities team to help them with their oxygen issues. It demonstrated the ability for health systems to come together and help each other, and Jamaica was in a critical position due to its oxygen delivery system. We had our facilities team reach out to discuss ways to address their oxygen supply issue. It's definitely a proud feeling to be able to help them."

* * *

One of the ways we kept the numbers in our emergency departments and inpatient units under control is that we were able to see seventy thousand patients in our Northwell Health-GoHealth Urgent Care Centers and many more patients in our other ambulatory locations. The GoHealth Urgent Care Centers, fifty-two in all, are spread throughout the greater New York area and treat non-life-threatening injuries and illnesses. Had we not had these urgent care centers, it is likely that a significant number of those seventy thousand patients would have shown up in our hospital emergency rooms. It would have been sheer mayhem. These facilities handled a record number of patients during the crisis when they were "completely inundated with sick people," said Adam Boll, vice president of joint venture operations. "Urgent care was one of the hardest hit components of our health system." Half of the seventy thousand were tested while the other half did not meet testing criteria. Of those who were tested, half proved to be infected with the virus. Fortunately, the great majority of the patients seen in the urgent care centers could be sent home to ride out the disease.

"We were able to serve as a de facto gatekeeping mechanism preventing all of these sick people from flooding our emergency rooms," he said. "I think that in itself was the biggest benefit to the health system. That GoHealth was able to take this brunt was pivotal because if we weren't able to do that, do the math: seventy thousand additional visits to our hospitals." These centers were so overwhelmed with patients that we had to redeploy staff from other parts of the system to help in urgent care. Many members of our GoHealth staff were infected. At the height of the pandemic, eleven of the fifty-two sites had to close due to illness among the staff. Tragically, one urgent care staff member, a retired New York City firefighter who had survived the 9/11 attack, was infected with the virus and passed away.

* * *

As Mark Solazzo said: "You need three things to care for patients in this crisis: Beds, equipment, and staff, and, by far, staff is the most important." All the beds and ventilators in the world won't help without the trained medical professionals to operate them and make judgments about how best to care for very sick and vulnerable patients.

As the crisis approached, it was clear that we did not have nearly enough frontline team members to care for the expected number of patients. We were about to handle ICU volumes far beyond anything we had ever experienced. There are a couple of components to the staff issue. One is that while we had enough "bodies," we didn't have enough of the specialists we needed given the nature of the virus. We needed more intensivists—doctors trained in the specialty of caring for patients in the intensive care unit—along with ICU nurses, emergency room primary care docs, respiratory therapists, pulmonary nurses, and others. There was an odd bit of good luck amid the crisis: Because we had to shut down our surgical units and many of our ambulatory sites, several thousand doctors and nurses who no longer had any work to do were freed up to help with COVID patients. We put out a call for help, asking clinical staff to take on new roles in our COVID units. Several hundred doctors, nurses, physician assistants, nurse practitioners, and others jumped in to help. Some specialists had skills immediately useful on the front lines. Pulmonologists, for example, typically have critical care training and could be redeployed to the ICU. Anesthesiologists are trained in managing patients on ventilators. Many physician assistants and nurse practitioners redeployed from orthopedic or ambulatory sites had prior experience working in hospital settings earlier in their careers. However, some of the staff newly available to help didn't have the current competencies to work in the areas needed. We conducted competency reviews and training for team members that were coming back to the bedside from procedural areas such as interventional radiology, cardiac catheterization lab, and perioperative services. In a way, everyone shifted in their specialty: Intensivists on the floor became "Covidists" while hospitalists (physicians who specialize in delivering care within a hospital) became intensivists and primary care docs became hospitalists. In the redeployment process, no one was cast into the deep end right away. We provided some basic training, including having our redeployed nonexpert staff shadow a doctor or nurse for a few days, and then found that fairly quickly these backup doctors and nurses, under supervision, were helping out in important ways.

These physician and nurse helpers allowed us to stretch the doctor-patient and nurse-patient ratios throughout our health system. The effect, as Dr. Lawrence Smith put it, was to "magnify the ability of a person

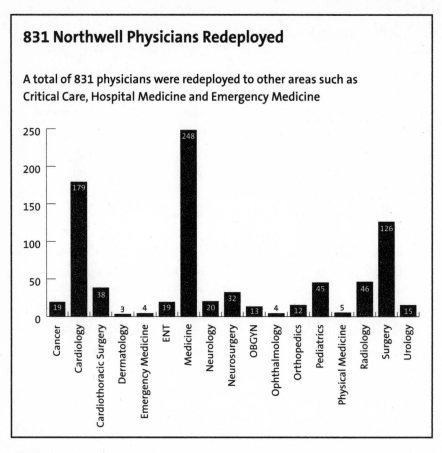

831 Northwell Physicians Redeployed

A total of 831 physicians were redeployed to other areas such as Critical Care, Hospital Medicine and Emergency Medicine

A total of 831 physicians were redeployed to other areas such as Critical Care, Hospital Medicine and Emergency Medicine.

who is an expert." Instead of having a critical care doctor for every five patients in the ICU, we would have one critical care doctor for the whole ICU with a number of other physicians with basic medical skills helping out. This allowed the experts to manage the sophisticated decisions that require in-depth knowledge of critical care.

Even with the redeployments, we were still short-staffed as the number of very sick patients continued to mount. One fact that helped was that our ICUs were transformed from places where very sick people suffered from a wide array of illnesses into a place where 90 percent of the patients suffered from exactly the same disease, meaning that virtually every patient required similar care. This simplified matters for doctors and nurses unaccustomed to a frontline role.

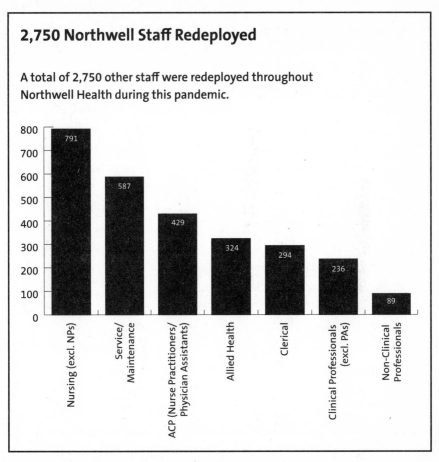

2,750 Northwell Staff Redeployed

A total of 2,750 other staff were redeployed throughout Northwell Health during this pandemic.

A total of 2,750 other staff were redeployed throughout Northwell Health during this pandemic.

A crucial development that helped with redeployment—that actually made it possible—was a declaration of emergency in New York State, which gave Governor Cuomo broad powers to suspend existing laws and regulations. Without this, there would have been chaos. The governor waived hundreds of rules and laws that would have prevented us from acting swiftly in the best interests of patients. For example, we needed help from doctors and nurses from other states. The governor waived the rule that requires licensure specifically in New York State. The state regulates where patients can be placed in a hospital. The governor waived that rule, which enabled us to increase capacity by placing beds in conference rooms, auditoriums, etc. And the governor provided legal protection from malpractice litigation for doctors not trained in intensive care medicine to work at the front lines. All of these rulings, and literally hundreds more, proved invaluable. Said Dr. Lawrence Smith:

> How can a dermatologist work as a backup physician in the medical ICU if he or she is open to getting sued for malpractice should he make a misjudgment in the heat of taking care of these patients? Because of course he's going to make some misjudgments. He or she never was trained in that specialty and so those [rulings from the state] were absolutely essential or nobody was going to do that. Nobody is going to say to you, "Listen, I am absolutely there. I'm going to help you with the epidemic. Of course, I realize that it is very likely I'm going to make some mistakes and I'll probably lose my house, my pension, everything I've ever worked for." Nobody is going to do this. They're going to say goodbye, I'll stay home. And those changes were absolutely essential to get anybody to do this.

* * *

In war, the saying goes that the Marines are the tip of the spear, leading the way headlong into enemy fire. It is fair to say that in the coronavirus crisis, the seventeen thousand nurses at Northwell Health were our Marines—the tip of the Northwell spear. And they were stretched thinner than just about any of them had ever experienced. Part of the problem, to start with, was that hundreds of nurses were infected with the virus and either out sick or forced to quarantine. At the peak, a total of 3,500 Northwell employees were out on furlough (full salary, full benefits, but unable to work) at one time as a result of COVID exposure or a positive test—it appeared the bulk of these infections came while employees were out in the community rather than working in the hospital. In early April, 425 registered nurses were out on quarantine, representing approximately 4 percent of the staff on that one day. Approximately 9 percent of staff RNs in total were diagnosed as positive between late February and the end of April. While all of our sites were impacted by team members going on furlough or on leave, some were hit harder than others. More than 20 percent of RNs at Forest Hills and Valley Stream were on a leave of absence at any point between March 1 and April 30.

When coupled with the explosion of patients entering our hospitals, staffing was an urgent priority requiring all hands on deck. On April 6, the average daily census throughout our system peaked at 46 percent above normal. Average daily census continued at above typical levels through April. To meet the increased patient demand, we would add more than 1,600 beds across our health system, and every one of those additional beds required additional staff.

In the planning stages we had anticipated a staff shortage, and Joe Moscola and Maureen White went out and contracted with national companies for traveling nurses, respiratory therapists, dialysis nurses, physicians' assistants, and nurse practitioners. "We wanted to be on the safe side and over-plan," said White. "We didn't know how many patients we would see or how long this would last. And it turned out that early

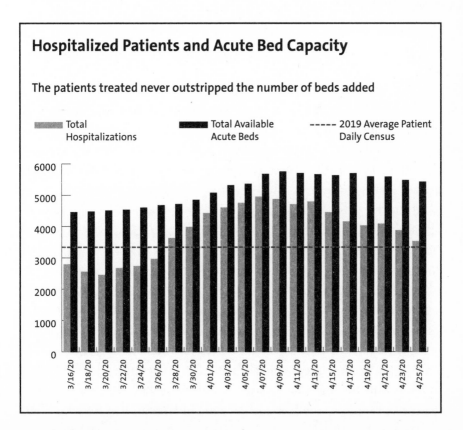

Hospitalized Patients and Acute Bed Capacity

The patients treated never outstripped the number of beds added planning was a Godsend." The travel nurses for whom we contracted came to us from all over the country, including Hawaii, California, Idaho, and everywhere in between. With help from our IT folks, we were able to train them when they were still at home on how to operate our electronic medical records. This was thanks in large measure to the nursing institute led by Maureen White.

In mid-February, before the virus arrived in our area, we reached out through an email system to all Northwell nurses who worked outside our hospitals either in offices or ambulatory sites, and let them know that with the virus headed our way we anticipated that we might need them at the bedside. To facilitate the reassignment process, we began to build labor pools not only of nurses but also of doctors and others who worked in our corporate offices or in our ambulatory sites. One element of the reassignment process was determining what role a team member could serve effectively and safely. This involved skill-testing corporate-based RNs and other team members eligible for reassignment who were no longer used to providing bedside care. "We weren't just saying, 'Go on in, you've got an 'RN' after your name and even though you haven't been at the bedside in fifteen years, you'll figure it out; it's like riding a bicycle,'" said Maureen White. "No, we took the time to prepare them, and we asked them, 'Do you think you can do this?' And it wasn't until they said, 'Yes, I can do this,' that they went to work." It was heartening how adaptable and flexible people were. Many clinicians who normally worked daytime hours volunteered for overnight or weekend shifts. The attitude among most people was: *I will do whatever you need me to do.* We asked these nurses to self-assess, as Maureen put it: "Are you somebody who could go back to the bedside and take a full patient care assignment because you only recently left? Are you somebody who left quite some time ago, but you'd be willing to go back to the bedside, take a smaller assignment, but you would need some competencies refreshed? Or are you somebody who really doesn't feel comfortable taking a patient care assignment, but could assist in patient care delivery under the direction of the primary nurse who was caring for however many patients?" The self-assessment also asked which nurses might be comfortable working as scribes for doctors on the electronic medical records. Requests for other volunteers went out to office staff who might have an EMT background, or were military veterans who might have been in the medical corps. In all, about 150 people from office staff positions throughout the system volunteered.

*   *   *

As much as we thought we had prepared, no one could prepare mentally or emotionally for the impact of dealing with such a volume of patients sick with a disease no one had ever successfully treated before. "I don't think any of us were mentally prepared for that volume at the pace at which it came," said White. "We knew we'd see a lot of patients; we've had a lot of patients during H1N1 and the different flu seasons, but there'd be a gradual build-up to the peak. There was no gradual build-up to this. You had one and then boom, now it's full-blown. I think that was different about this emergency than other emergencies that I'd been through."

The nature of the disease was new and shocking to nurses and doctors and for about the first ten days or so many nurses were quite uncomfortable dealing with the crisis. But nurses are a resilient breed, and it was clear that they gained confidence after a couple of weeks' worth of experience. You could sense a rise in confidence throughout our system. Nurses were saying basically, *yes, this is new and frightening, but we know what to do. We've got this.* Simple innovations helped a lot. Nurses were protected in stations where there was a closed door between them and the patient. The fewer trips a nurse made into a patient room the safer he or she would be. That led many of our sites to use iPads at the patient's bedside that could be monitored centrally. One hospital, when iPads were unavailable, used baby monitors borrowed from the OB suites! This allowed nurses to keep eyes and ears on the patient while going into the room only when necessary.

*   *   *

Among the toughest challenges for nurses was dealing with fear. The fear eased somewhat once we were past the peak and the caseload began to decline. But even then there were still many patients who came in, seemed all right at the start, and then tumbled downhill on to ventilators. Many of those patients did not survive. The speed of the demise of patients made nurses understandably fearful for themselves, even when they felt just fine. The reality was that they had seen many patients who seemed fine one day and were intubated the next.

As White reflects on the crisis, she believes that the early commitment from our organization to sign contracts with travel nurses and our recruitment of other nurses from within our system were lifesaving moves. At the same time, she believes that we could have done a better job preparing nurses for what was to come. We didn't anticipate the landslide; the unprecedented crush of very sick patients. White and other nurse leaders said nurses should expect a significant increase in the workload, but the reality was an order of magnitude beyond that. "Intellectually, they understood what we were saying," said White, "but when it really came down to, 'Oh my goodness, I really have to take care of that many patients,' it was very difficult for them to adjust. It was very overwhelming for them." They were used to doing all the work themselves and now they had to work with a helper, what we referred to as a functional nurse. And the lead nurses had to learn on the fly how to decide which work to do themselves and which tasks to delegate to their helpers. They were forced to learn an entirely new management skill in the midst of the worst crisis we had ever experienced. "The patients came so fast that they couldn't get their heads around it," she said.

In the crisis, everything was stressful, even having to don and doff PPE. Nurses at a central station in a hallway could communicate with patients via iPads, but when a nurse needed to go into a patient room, he or she put on a gown, gloves, booties, a face mask, and protective goggles or protective face shields over the face mask. Hand washing prior to entry into the room was required and then again afterward. The face shield and goggles had to be disinfected. But logistical preparation with PPE was one thing. Quite another was the emotional preparation for so much sickness and death, and the randomness of it, and the powerlessness of not being able to save person after person after person and the fear that generated. How could anyone prepare for that?

In retrospect, White said, she should have guided the frontline teams to a greater sense of introspection and clarity about handling double the caseload before the onslaught. Nurse leaders should have thought about ways to ease the burden, she said. For example, they might have reduced the amount of documentation required or eliminated certain types of rounds. "I think it would have mentally prepared them more for that worst-case scenario instead of us just kind of telling them at a high level, 'Oh, now, it's ballooning.' I think it would have helped them to walk a little bit more in the reality, if they had been part of that planning process."

* * *

For all that we did, we remained under pressure to find additional staff. While the voluntary approach worked well, we found as the crisis deepened that the caseload threatened to overwhelm us. Thus, we were forced to issue a mandatory redeployment order. The policy required employees to accept whatever new role was assigned to them, and most did exactly that. Workers who declined the reassignment could take up to seven days of paid time off after which the employee would go on unpaid leave (though with full benefits maintained) for an indefinite period. This was a tough policy and not everyone was happy about it. There were workers who felt vulnerable themselves or were concerned about bringing the infection home to their families—in some cases, aging parents or grandparents. Dr. Thomas McGinn was approached by physicians who objected to redeployment from a safe specialty to the front lines. "They would say to me, 'I've got a sick mother at home,' or 'I'm nervous because my kids are at home,' and I would say, 'Let me introduce you to my chief of the ICU who's there every day. She's got grandparents at home and four young children.'"

The greatest internal conflict within our health system during the pandemic involved employees who wanted accommodations related to redeployment. The problem was that with several thousand employees infected with the virus, our workforce was depleted just at a time when we needed to expand the talent pool. The reality—how could it be otherwise—was that fear spread through the provider community like a virus itself. Dr. Mark Jarrett put it this way:

When you have a mass casualty incident or something like 9/11 or the Boston Marathon bombing, those are horrific events, but for caregivers once it's over they are no longer at risk. With the pandemic, we are all at risk. When you see a colleague who's sick with it or maybe even passes away from it, it actually reminds you of your own mortality and the risk to you and your family. Everybody is scared. People are right to be scared because, really, you don't have any proven treatments. It has been so random. We talk all the time about the elderly and immune-compromised, but the reality is we're unfortunately seeing young, healthy people who have gotten extremely ill, or passed away. That becomes scary and stressful to our staff.

"If you made accommodations for all who are considered at risk in this disease, you would easily wipe out upwards of half of the workforce," said Joe Moscola. "We'd never be able to meet the surge needs." Exempting older workers, pregnant women and spouses, and workers with cancer or chronic conditions, you would eliminate an estimated fifteen thousand people from the workforce. Accommodations went to high-risk individuals who had preexisting conditions that placed them at elevated risk. Some of these folks were reassigned to the call center or other office duty. Still other employees simply said they were too concerned about the virus to work and would opt for a leave of absence. As Moscola put it: "If you don't feel comfortable, we understand." There were suggestions that anyone refusing redeployment should be fired, but that made no sense to Moscola. He focused on the big picture, which included the monumental task of reopening the health system post-COVID, and that reopening would require the efforts of every employee. In the end, very few employees chose the furlough route. "Ninety-five percent of the doctors helped," said McGinn. "Some go through a process, talk it over for a little while, and there's a small percentage that just can't do it. They just can't. And I don't judge them. I get it."

Dr. David Battinelli acknowledged that this has been a difficult experience for many doctors and nurses, but he also argued that this is what they signed up for in the first place. "So, now you have all these people who went into health care and might've been in health care for a long time, since the last big thing that came about, which was HIV in the early eighties," said Battinelli. "And we had a very similar response then. But since that time—that's a long time ago, almost forty years ago—and you've got a whole bunch of people choosing careers in medicine where there really wasn't a chance you were going to get sick." He heard some people say, they 'didn't sign up for this.' Not so fast, he said. "My view is, 'well, what did you think you signed up for?' That's like the military guys saying, you know, 'I want to be in the reserves, because it's probably a cool time. I'll put my years in, I'll take my pension, blah, blah, blah. I hope there's not a war.' And then when the war comes, they're saying they didn't sign up for this. Yes, you actually did sign up for this. You were hoping it wasn't going to happen, but that is what you signed up for."

* * *

We learned an important lesson about redeployment. We would have been much better prepared if we'd had a data base that would quickly tell us which members of our staff had recent clinical experience. Instead of having that data readily available, we had to comb through electronic files and reach out to ask people the question. We have already started building precisely that type of data base in preparation for next time. "It wasn't as clear who was available on the bench from all the practices that were shuttered," said Dr. D'Angelo. "Who were the people that had physician notes that said because of their underlying medical conditions they couldn't work in a COVID environment or they couldn't work in a hospital anymore? I think we probably could have been a little bit more organized initially in knowing who could be redeployed where and how and what the limitations were. It could have been orchestrated: who is available to redeploy and when."

Despite this shortcoming, and given the reality that hundreds of our workers each day were exposed to the virus, the redeployment worked well and we can say with confidence that it saved lives. There was a price to pay, however, in the form of psychological impact on staff. We had counselors and chaplains spread out at our sites, especially those hardest hit by the virus. Some staff opened up and shared their anxieties and sought reassurance. Others remained stoic. We worked to try and prevent PTSD among staff, but we are sure more and more will surface in the time ahead. It is not dissimilar to the military where combatants see terrible things even as they continue on with their mission, only to suffer psychologically many months or even years later.

* * *

As we look back and reflect on the crisis, it is clear that the incident command structure played a crucial role in our ability to get through. So, too, did the size of our system and our load-balancing capabilities. But ultimately the people answering the call of duty made the difference. In the words of Kevin Beiner, senior vice president and regional executive director, "People didn't show up to work anymore. They came to do a more profound job. They came to answer a call, and every one of them, from the moment they opened their eyes in the morning until the moment they closed them at night, they were working." They were attending bedsides, shipping supplies, moving patients, gathering data, counseling on the phone, and coordinating plans. Throughout the crisis, few leaders within the system had a day off, and you haven't heard a single complaint about that. Beiner continued his thought:

> People are certainly weary, but you haven't heard a complaint. And I think it comes from two or three things. I think it's this constant alignment to what we're here for and the selection of people that know that they're here for a higher purpose. I think it's also because people like each other. And they answered a duty not mechanically but emotionally and they did their jobs.
>
> Some people are here for the money. Some people are here for power or whatever the reason is, but I've always felt that given the difficulty of the decisions that we have to make on a regular basis and the challenges inherent in this industry, you have to see something bigger in it. If not, I'm not sure what your path is going to be, but I think we've selected leaders that mostly see that. They mostly get the higher calling. We're here

not just for the patients or for the communities, but also we're here for each other. I think it's kind of a beautiful thing, that it causes people to put themselves second. I've watched people risk their own lives, the lives of their families, to come in and do what it is that they do. I'm glad to have seen it. I hope never to have to see it again, but certainly over an extended period it's a pretty awesome human thing to watch.

CHAPTER FOUR

Staff Safety and Morale

Lessons
- In order to care for patients, the top priority must be protecting the health and safety of staff.
- Staff members must be protected physically with sufficient quantities of PPE and have the knowledge that there will always be sufficient supplies.
- Staff members must be protected emotionally through the availability of active employee assistance programs that provide on-site counseling.
- Tranquility tents allow frontline workers to calm themselves as they reflect, meditate, or pray before or after shifts.
- Leaders must demonstrate through communication and via personal presence at the front lines that the work of employees is valued and that staff safety is the highest management priority.
- Prepare to have employee assistance personnel, including counselors and chaplains, readily available when a frontline staff member passes away.

North Shore University Hospital is the largest of the twenty-three Northwell hospitals. Located in Manhasset, New York, it includes 766 beds and employs more than six thousand staff members, including four thousand physicians working in a wide array of medical specialties.

North Shore is a sprawling facility spread out over a fifty-seven-acre campus, with twenty-three operating rooms where every conceivable kind of surgery is performed, including the transplantation of livers, kidneys, and hearts. Much of the business at North Shore involves previously scheduled surgeries. Some are elective—a new knee or hip, or plastic surgery. Many others are medically necessary but not emergencies. At North Shore we are known in particular for our cardiac and neurological procedures. Hundreds of patients are scheduled each day with bookings taking place weeks or even months in advance. But with the virus bearing down, it was necessary to clear the schedule of all but the most urgent cases in order to open beds for COVID patients. Canceling thousands of scheduled cases was no small matter, but we got it done.

Our first COVID patient arrived at North Shore on March 7. By March 14 we had sixty patients, and five days later we had nearly 150. Two and a half to three weeks in, that number climbed to a census of four hundred patients very sick from the virus, and our projections indicated there would be many hundreds more, perhaps thousands more, headed our way. In all, we cared for 2,492 COVID patients at North Shore. Thus, we were racing to add bed capacity, a pursuit Tara Laumenede, acting chief nursing officer, likened to laying track in front of a moving train. Laumenede and her team identified opportunities to consolidate and flip units to COVID care quickly. They also moved all the patients around and staffed the units.

As the teams at North Shore converted many areas of the facility into beds for COVID patients, it was suggested that the cafeteria should be converted to a patient area. But Jon Sendach, head of the hospital, said no. "Once you do that, there's no place for your employees to get away from the units," he said. "And that's when it would feel to them as if this is not the hospital they work in, and there's an emotional component to that." Sendach's view was that staff members need a place they can go to take a deep breath, get a cup of coffee or a sandwich, and chat with their coworkers. Sendach would do whatever he could to protect the cafeteria for his workers.

As we have said before and will say again, caring for the safety and morale of our frontline staff was our number one priority and we did it in many different ways. We focus in this chapter on the efforts at North Shore University Hospital, but comparable efforts to care for staff needs were spread throughout our system. Jon Sendach and Dr. Michael Gitman, chief medical officer at North Shore, and their executive team recognized during the surge planning that it was important to protect the cafeteria as a refuge for staff. And Sendach went a bit further. He not only kept it open, he went to the culinary staff—"we have unbelievable culinary talent here"—and asked them to start putting together whole meals to go for employees. There were meals for two, four, even for families of eight packaged up—including plates, utensils, and napkins—and ready to go as staff members left work for the night. For staff who did not want premade meals, Sendach had the cafeteria team open what amounted to a small grocery store where staff could buy vegetables, fruits, meats, etc., without having to stop at the supermarket on the way home and risk possible contamination.

It seemed a small thing, but it was meaningful to staff and it was the kind of gesture that was consistent with how the organization had been treating employees under the HR leadership of Joseph Moscola. Moscola had made so many improvements in how staff members were treated and rewarded that, in 2019, Northwell was named one of the *Fortune Magazine* top hundred best companies to work for—a huge accomplishment. That hard-won designation would be put to the test in the crisis in terms of how well we were able to protect the physical and emotional well-being of our staff. Baseline safety required ample supplies of PPE. What did that mean exactly? It meant that we had to provide all of the PPE staff needed whenever they needed it. But it also meant establishing policies such as requiring masks of all patients in the ED, before any other system did so. Eventually, we required all employees across all parts of the hospital to wear masks.

In an atmosphere of unprecedented fear and anxiety, it was important to care for the emotional needs of our people as well. Employees need to know that their well-being is the top priority for the hospital's leadership. They need to see their leaders with them, encouraging them at the front lines. Our employees talked about an article in the *New York Post* about the leader of another health system who chose to remain in Florida when the crisis broke. Our workers were putting their health and the health of their loved ones on the line, and they needed to know every shift that we were with them and doing everything possible to keep them safe.

A key element of safety is for the people running our individual facilities to know that senior executives at our corporate offices have their back. Joe Moscola and Dr. Mark Jarrett realized very early on that once staff members started getting sick the organization would fall behind, and that there could be a domino effect from staff falling too ill to work. Working in partnership with chief nursing executive Maureen White, Moscola managed the flow of staff throughout the system, contracted for hundreds of additional workers from around the country, and put in place a series of initiatives that supported the physical and psychological needs of employees. The HR team:

- established staffing standards across the system so that the professional competence of each worker matched his or her assignment;
- contracted to house thousands of our employees in dozens of hotels to support workers who did not want to go home for fear of infecting their families;
- deployed professionals from our employee assistance program to our facilities where they were readily available to meet with staff to talk through concerns and fears and in some cases to refer staff for additional counseling;
- set up what were known as *tranquility tents* so that workers going into or leaving a shift could sit calmly and reflect, meditate, or pray. The tents proved helpful to some of our workers for whom a brief period of calm reflection supported them in getting through the day;
- made sure staff members were well fed and that there were open lines to HR for any staff member with a concern of any kind.

* * *

In late March, word came that our health system had been able to purchase another large supply of N95 masks from 3M. This required everyone on the front lines at North Shore to be fit-tested for the mask, a process that went on around the clock for several days until everyone needing such a mask had the proper fit. Meanwhile, Sendach was tightening

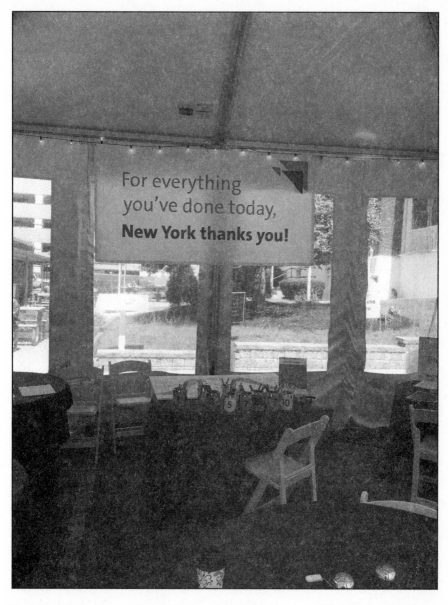

For everything
you've done today,
New York thanks you!

The tranquility tents provided staff a needed respite from the stress of constant patient care in their units.

procedures to keep workers safer. He announced a plan to reduce the number of times doctors and nurses would have to enter a patient's room. The clinical team extended IV tubing to reach out into the hallway outside a room so staff in the hall could check on the IV drip. IT helped clinicians monitor patient rooms via iPads and cell phones.

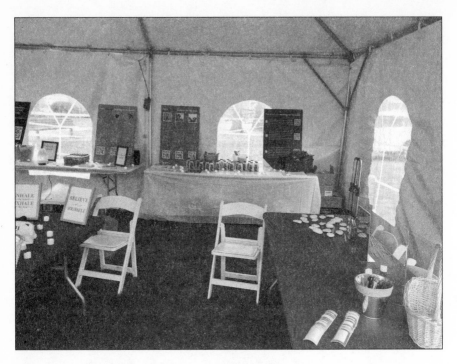

The tents provided ample opportunities to reduce stress and promote well-being.

In February, Sendach and colleagues joined a call with hospital leaders in Italy when the Italians were going through hell: "They told us that 'it's going to trickle and then, by the second week, it's going to just overwhelm you.' They told us it's not exclusively older people; that they were not sure why people crashed so suddenly." And they issued a warning: Unless you take steps to protect them, you will lose 20 percent of your staff to illness, which would require them to quarantine. Throughout our health system there was a mix of emotions as we worked to prepare for the virus. Yes, it was true that we had prepared well. We had leaders who believed deeply in the culture of emergency preparedness that is such a fundamental part of our identity. But we are human beings, and the horrors from China and Italy were frightening. Would we be able to handle it? Were we as good at this type of work as we thought we were? Or were we guilty of excessive pride, of the kind of hubris that brings one crashing down?

* * *

Sendach was a classic Northwell executive. He had started working in the system in the back of an ambulance as an EMT, and like so many others in our system, he loves emergency work. After getting his Master of Public Administration degree, he moved up in management ranks, to the point where he runs our largest hospital. For the 2020 spring semester, he was teaching a course on health-care management at the Wagner Graduate School of Public Service at NYU. "The course was on leading change for executives," he said, and in that course he talked about the need to respond to challenging circumstances, including emergencies. "And I said to myself when all this started, 'well, you know what? You're about to find out if you actually know how to do it.'"

The initiative to protect staff started in the emergency department where sick patients congregated, some shedding virus in the vicinity of staff members. The ED clinical team worked to get patients moved into, through, and out of the ED as expeditiously as possible on the theory that the less time sick patients spent in the vicinity of ED employees, the safer those workers. Sendach had seen pictures and video of hospitals in New York City—notably Elmhurst—where the emergency department was overrun, frontline workers inundated with highly contagious patients. "We could not let the ER get overrun here," he said. "We just made a commitment that we were going to have an operationalized team so that when patients were brought in, once evaluated, we would whisk them out of the ER as quickly as we could up to the units and those extra beds. Because once it backs up in the ER, then you end up in a situation where that workforce gets sick and infected and you start getting into a situation where emotionally, they feel as though they're wide open, that no one's protecting them."

A similar threat existed with nurses in open spaces where new beds had been installed. This was the case in some recovery areas. Nurses at a station in the vicinity of a dozen ICU patients would be vulnerable. There would be no doors to close between the nurses and the patients, and the virus would be swirling in the air around the nurses. "What is our message to you as an employee if we allow that to happen?" Sendach asked. Sendach got the engineering team in to build walls around the makeshift nursing stations and pump purified air into that space. These enclosures were not pretty—"they look kind of like prisons," said Sendach—but they protected the staff. "You cannot ask people to sit there for twelve hours, even with their N95s on, in an environment where they don't feel remotely protected."

On the calls to Italy, the Italian doctors had warned of potential harm from aerosolizing the virus. This was a serious problem for clinical staff in close contact with COVID patients. A clinician intubating a patient would pass a tube down the throat causing many patients to cough or gag, sending streams of virus into the air directly at the clinician. No matter how well gowned and masked workers were, this was a hostile environment. Once again, the engineering shop came to the rescue. There was a picture online from Taiwan of a Plexiglas box that looked like a square helmet that a Martian might wear. By placing it over the patient's head, the clinician could then reach through arm holes and perform the intubation protected from the spray of virus. At North Shore, the idea of using such devices was proposed by Kelly Treacy, the nurse executive in charge of the operating rooms. Treacy proposed the idea on Monday, March 23. She discussed it with anesthesiologist Dr. Rich Grieco that day and the next. They engaged two outside vendors to design four prototypes. Early on Thursday, March 26, Treacy, Grieco,

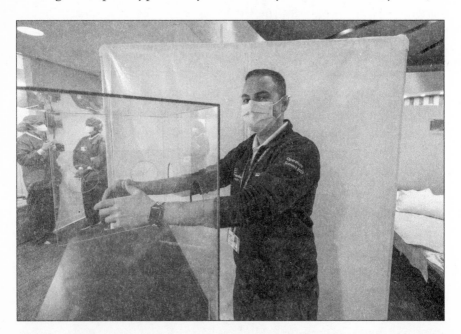

This is an example of the Plexiglas box used for patients at North Shore University Hospital.

and a number of other clinicians reviewed the design, offered a few modifications, and by Friday completed devices were arriving at the hospital. Over the next two weeks twelve devices were built internally in our workshop while an additional seventy-five were manufactured externally and distributed throughout the Northwell system. The last step was to post the device's CAD drawings on an open-source site so that anybody could copy it.

* * *

During the crisis, the availability of PPE was *the* issue for staff. Without the proper equipment, how could they possibly come to work and do their jobs? The availability of protective material for the staff is key to staff engagement and morale because they're worried about their safety, and legitimately so. At a certain point, Sendach saw that "there was constant nonsense back and forth about masks and gowns on the units and which unit was running out and who was hoarding and who was grabbing an extra box." Sendach's colleague Will Corrigan, associate executive director for hospital operations, had a solution: Set up a PPE station at the entrance where employees arrived for their shift. "So, when you come into work through our team entrance, we have someone handing you snacks to make your shift that much better. And the next thing you walk past is a huge PPE depot. *You need a mask? You need a gown? You need more gloves? Whatever you need, no questions asked. Please, stop right here.* And we'd just feed the depot instead of having staff members running around delivering boxes and boxes and boxes up to units."

Sendach wanted to know about any concerns on the part of the staff; any fears about unsafe working conditions. To find out what was on the minds of employees and to inspect working conditions throughout the facility, Sendach created a small team of inspectors led by the chair of emergency medicine, the vice chair of surgery, and a RN. These men and women wore bright teal vests upon which were printed *Healthcare Personnel Safety Team.* They would check in with employees—*hey, how's your mask? Your gowns? Any questions about what you should be doing with your masks and gowns?* Sendach wanted employees to know without any doubt that there was a major effort being undertaken to protect them.

At the peak, there were 715 COVID patients at North Shore, which made the hospital one of the largest COVID specialty facilities in the United States. At the same time we were caring for more than a hundred patients with conditions other than COVID who needed urgent or emergency care, including lifesaving surgeries. We kept these patients secure in non-COVID areas of the campus. In all, at the peak, Sendach had a total of nine hundred beds available with the ability to push it all the way up to 1,200 had it been necessary.

In mid-April, North Shore had 150 COVID-positive patients in the ICU on ventilators. These patients would end up staying for close to

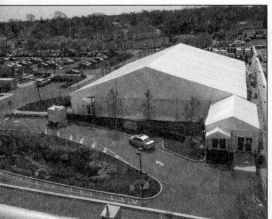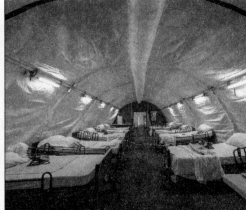

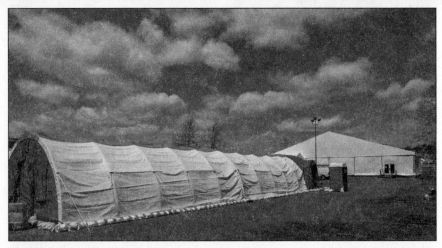

The external mobile tents were just an example of the many alternative treatment areas created during the height of the crisis.

three weeks on average. Most would not make it. It was another one of the surreal things happening in the time of this pandemic. Normally, patients who are intubated spend a bit of time on the ventilator and are then extubated and recover. With the virus, however, during the crisis an estimated 60 percent of ventilated patients did not survive. Such a tragedy, Sendach thought, families losing a spouse, parent, sibling, grandparent and in some cases, God forbid, a child.

Sendach and Dr. Gitman, the North Shore chief medical officer, work closely together, and Sendach watched as Gitman had one conversation after another with physicians and family members about decisions in treating patients. "What do we do about intubating, not intubating, talking about Do Not Resuscitate, trying to withdraw care on patients?" asked Sendach. There were many difficult decisions doctors had to make, said Sendach, "ethical choices and decisions about patient care. Is there a medical benefit to putting another person on a ventilator so that they can then spend three or four weeks on it and have a poor prognosis? It's just staggering."

On a Saturday in mid-April, Sendach joined in a North Shore celebration for the one thousandth COVID patient discharged from the

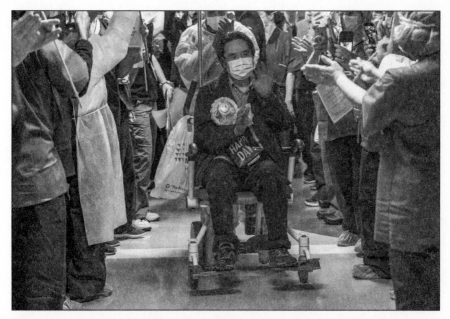

Pictured is the thousandth patient discharged from North Shore University Hospital.

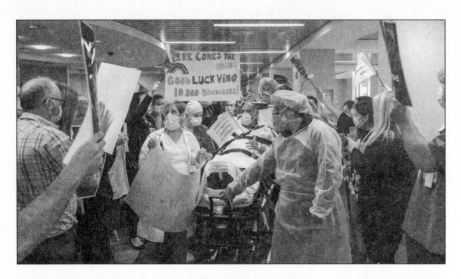

It was not long before the ten thousandth patient was discharged from Northwell Health.

hospital. Celebrating success turned out to be important throughout our system. It was brutal for doctors and nurses to have so many patients on ventilators dying. When patients did survive and were able to go home from the hospital, it was time for celebration. "Leaders have to be celebrators," said Dr. McGinn. "You've got to celebrate heroics and you've got to celebrate success. And you've got to do it very consistently. We're constantly thanking people and creating camaraderie and when any patient gets off a respirator, we try to make time to celebrate that and highlight that." McGinn and other doctors have been impressed with the level of camaraderie among the frontline doctors, nurses, respiratory therapists, transporters, cleaning crews, food service workers, and on and on.

The celebration of the one thousandth discharged patient was a happy occasion for the patients, families, and staff. And when it took place, in mid-April, there was also a growing sense that the crisis was just beginning to ease in the New York area. On April 15, Sendach and Dr. Gitman wrote to the North Shore staff:

> We are seeing an increase in the number of patients going home and those who progress toward recovery. It is critical that we balance that against the growing number who require critical care and advanced respiratory support. We understand for those of you actively on the frontlines and at the bedside,

the news outside may at times feel incongruent with your perspective. Our hope is that in the coming days, the positive impact on what has now been a ten-day trend of slightly lower ED volume and resultant hospitalizations will be felt in a softening of our census throughout the hospital. We all feel better each time we hear those chimes overhead, announcing another patient has been discharged . . .

Yesterday we had the opportunity to visit several units with a small crew from CBS News . . . and were again reminded what an incredible spirit exists here. For a short piece that aired this morning on *CBS This Morning* . . . the producer and reporter . . . told us as they left that they came here to cover a story of crisis at a major medical center in the county that now has the most cases of any county in the nation outside of New York City. Their visit forced them to change their story line somewhat. What they reported this morning was that they found a place where professional people are managing a crisis with class and a sense of calm purpose.

Despite the celebrations, Sendach also realized the toll the disease had taken. The same weekend as the discharge ceremony, thirty patients at North Shore died from the virus. At North Shore, our teams took care of thousands of COVID patients and never got overwhelmed. The teams laying track managed to stay well enough ahead of the roaring locomotive that was the virus. This was a victory as well as a relief. After the calls with the Italians, Sendach hadn't been sure what was coming exactly. Nobody was. At the worst point during the crisis, hundreds of North Shore staff members were out sick with the virus. By mid-April that was down to 1 percent, an impressive accomplishment given that at Forest Hills, at the peak, 6 percent of the workforce was out with the virus.

* * *

One other aspect of employee morale relies on the actions of the most senior executives in the health system. At Northwell, for example, our chief nursing executive, Maureen White, invested time walking the wards, encouraging the nursing staff, engaging in conversation, listening, and commiserating. Typically, nurses work in a crowded, bustling environment with patients' visitors often crowding hallways and patient rooms. But all of that visitor traffic was gone now and it was an oddly freeing thing for nurses to be able to move around without any interference. At the same time, many missed the human contact with families.

With so little human contact, it became especially meaningful when our senior executive leaders made a point of visiting units and spending time talking with nurses and doctors. Many of our senior physicians—Drs. David Battinelli, Mark Jarrett, John D'Angelo, Lawrence Smith, and Thomas McGinn—did this. Perhaps most notable was the presence at the front lines of one of us (Michael Dowling), who made it a point during the crisis period to go to the front lines, walk the wards, and encourage staff in the ICUs and emergency departments. During many of these sessions, nurses would ask to have photographs taken. These clinical and administrative leaders initially found nurses and doctors virtually unidentifiable as they were buried under layers of PPE. Then many

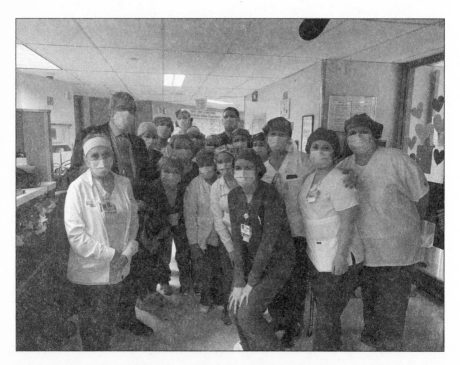

Pictured here is Michael Dowling meeting with nursing staff at Mather Hospital.

began to scrawl their first names on the outside of their PPE. And then a great trend among many nurses started —they blew up pictures from their ID badges and displayed them on the front of their PPE – a nice humanizing touch in an intimidating atmosphere.

It is hard to describe how great these frontline workers were. We tried throughout to demonstrate our gratitude to them. We did it in many ways and one especially meaningful action we took was to provide a bonus of $2,500 to every frontline employee, along with an additional week of paid vacation. For our staff members who tragically passed away, we continued to pay full salary to the family for an additional six months, and we covered all funeral expenses. We held a major internal fundraiser with all funds directed to the surviving families. And we have constructed a beautiful memorial honoring those who died in front of our main office. These were tangible ways to express our gratitude.

* * *

Keeping employees safe meant they were better able to meet the complex needs of our patients. COVID patients were not only very sick, but they were also separated from loved ones. One of the key questions for our patient experience team was to figure out how to create a human connection. It was not only COVID patients, but all our patients who were isolated and cut off from the outside world. Our only option was to do whatever was necessary to set up virtual visits for patients and their families.

"We couldn't get enough devices into the buildings fast enough, so we worked very closely with IT to break some rules to make sure that we did the right thing for the patients," said Sven Gierlinger, chief experience officer. We had been focused on using Android-based tablets for security reasons in part because the data from a very private visit between patient and family was wiped clean. Unlike Apple's iPad, with an Android, "there's no information left on the device." A nurse asked Gierlinger to waive the Android rule but he said he was unable to do so for security reasons. "When I told her that she said, 'that's really a shame and that's really tragic because I have now a family driving down from upstate New York to see their family member. And they're probably not going to make it in time. They're in the car right now. We can't do a Skype session with them or anything else. All they have is FaceTime and we have to do FaceTime."

Gierlinger knew they had to change the policy immediately. He went to John Bosco, head of IT, and said that we have a moral responsibility to enable the family to connect via FaceTime. Bosco totally understood, and right away enabled the technology so that the family could have their final words together. "It was gut-wrenching and a beautiful thing at the same time," said Gierlinger.

CHAPTER FIVE

Protecting the Supply Lifeline

Lessons
- A competent and effective internal supply-chain infrastructure with experienced leadership is essential.
- Strong relationships with vendors, built and nurtured over many years, are lifesaving in the midst of a crisis.
- It is dangerous to continue an over-reliance on China or any other country for the manufacture of essential supplies and equipment. There is an urgent need for domestic manufacturing capabilities.
- The state and federal governments should take a leadership role in stockpiling PPE without undermining the ability of health systems and hospitals to do the same.
- Allow staff to be creative in addressing problems that can be solved immediately. Internal innovation capabilities will surprise you.

On Monday, January 13, 2020, Phyllis McCready knew there was something wrong with the supply chain for the precious PPE frontline workers relied upon. McCready had been in this line of work for thirty years, ten at Columbia Presbyterian Medical Center and twenty at Northwell. Through years of dealing with hundreds of different vendors of medical equipment and supplies—beds, ventilators, PPE, oxygen, syringes, etc.—she had developed a keen instinct. She knew the business inside and out; knew the companies she could rely upon to ship exactly what she wanted when she wanted it; and knew the companies to avoid. She knew how much equipment she needed in the Northwell warehouse and she knew how much of just about any supply she would need in the next week or month or year.

But on January 13 her world changed when her instinct told her there was a serious problem at the manufacturing end of the supply chain in China. While we purchased supplies manufactured in a number of countries, the overwhelming majority were made in China. On that Monday morning, McCready got word that there was something not quite right with an order from her largest supplier, Cardinal Health. Cardinal is an American-owned multinational health services company so central to the medical supply chain that 90 percent of US hospitals are customers. Cardinal notified McCready that a shipment of surgical procedure packs from China had been compromised. Procedure packs are preassembled sets of sterile supplies such as syringes, surgical gowns, drapes, sponges, skin markers, suction catheters, and more, all needed for surgery. Having everything in one pack saves staff from having to collect a number of individual supplies. The representative from Cardinal told McCready that there was a problem specifically with the surgical gown in the pack. "He said that the surgical gown in the pack was compromised," recalled McCready, "and I said, 'Okay, since the pack is sterilized in the United States that's not a problem. We can take the gown out of the pack and we can use everything else.' And he said, 'No, you can't use the pack at all.'"

McCready pressed the representative from Cardinal, but he didn't seem to have answers. He promised to get back to McCready with more information. A couple of hours later he called and told McCready that not only was there a problem with the gown, but that Cardinal was not going to be able to ship any of the packs that McCready had ordered at all. McCready pressed the representative again, but he had little information. To McCready, this was unthinkable. How could this possibly happen? The doctors and nurses at Northwell hospitals needed this equipment in order to care for patients. Cardinal's representative told her that there was a "process problem" in the plant and that everything was on hold.

This was mystifying. What did that even mean, *process problem*? In all her years working in the field, McCready had never heard of a so-called process problem. After multiple calls with Cardinal's upper management over the week, she still wasn't getting any answers. "We never had a recall of this magnitude from a national company like Cardinal," she said. "No notification. They just stopped shipping. It was strange to me, and I kept saying to my team, 'Something is wrong.' I even reached out to the FDA trying to get information about Cardinal packs and the recall, and I got none. This was a major recall; this was a nightmare. That day, I panicked," she continued. "That was the first day in my career that I panicked. This is a major problem and not only for us, but for everyone." McCready was well-prepared for almost anything—hurricane, flood, blackout, etc. But this was different. "I felt like I wasn't ready," she said. "I wasn't prepared for this."

* * *

It is no small irony that the products and supplies that would soon be desperately needed in the United States to protect clinicians from COVID-19 were actually manufactured in Wuhan, China, where it is believed the virus originated. In mid-January coronavirus alarms had not yet been sounded in the United States, but the process problem with that Cardinal shipment had McCready's alarms ringing loudly. "That incident gave me a glimpse of what was happening in China," she said. "The problem with Cardinal was very suspicious to me, because they never really told me what the issue was." Evidently the gowns within the packs had been compromised in some way and the FDA would not permit release of the products. This was a very big deal in the US market and amplified McCready's sense of alarm.

"It was a very uncomfortable time," she recalled. She was hearing news out of Wuhan about people getting sick, and she saw Chinese New Year coming when people would be together spreading the virus, and she pulled her team together and told them it looked like the makings of a perfect storm. She feared a tighter squeeze in the pipeline out of China and dreaded the prospect that it could conceivably shut down altogether. She instructed the staff to go out and buy as many Chinese-manufactured

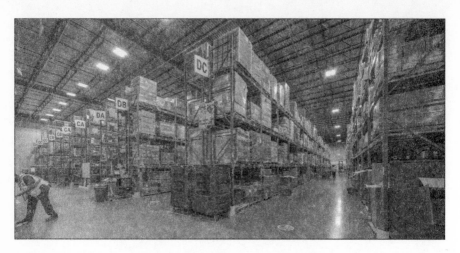

Pictured here is our internal distribution center in Bethpage, New York.

supplies as possible. She put in large orders for scrubs, gloves, bouffant caps, isolation gowns, shoe covers, procedural masks, disposable lab coats, face shields, and more. She called another major supplier, Medtronic, and said: "We need supplies and we need them now."

In purchasing equipment and supplies at Northwell, we have some built-in advantages. Because our system is so large, we make bulk purchases that vendors prefer. In addition, a decade ago, we established our own Group Purchasing Organization (GPO) and we store huge quantities of supplies in our Long Island warehouse. This Amazon-like automated warehouse is staffed by teams who distribute thousands of supplies to locations throughout our system. As the pandemic approached New York, we had a good supply of PPE in the warehouse along with strong relationships with our vendors, both domestic and international.

Through the rest of January and into February, McCready and her team, working with Northwell's Senior Vice President Donna Drummond, continued to focus on getting as much material from China as possible for fear of an imminent break in the supply chain. Not only were thousands of medical products manufactured there; many products manufactured elsewhere relied upon raw material produced in China. The over-reliance on Chinese production for the medical supply chain came into sharp relief during the crisis. One of the major lessons we learned is that, going forward, we will need a more diverse and reliable

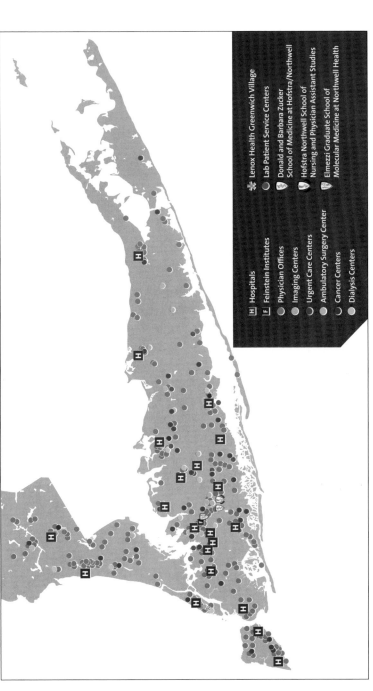

Legend:

- Ⓗ Hospitals
- Ⓕ Feinstein Institutes
- ● Physician Offices
- ● Imaging Centers
- ● Urgent Care Centers
- ● Ambulatory Surgery Center
- ◑ Cancer Centers
- ● Dialysis Centers
- ✱ Lenox Health Greenwich Village
- ● Lab Patient Service Centers
- 🎓 Donald and Barbara Zucker School of Medicine at Hofstra/Northwell
- 🎓 Hofstra Northwell School of Nursing and Physician Assistant Studies
- 🎓 Elmezzi Graduate School of Molecular Medicine at Northwell Health

Northwell Health is New York State's largest health care provider and private employer, with 23 hospitals, nearly 800 outpatient facilities, and more than 14,200 affiliated physicians. We care for over two million people annually in the New York metro area and beyond, thanks to philanthropic support from our communities. Our 72,000 employees—17,000-plus nurses and 4,500 employed doctors, including members of Northwell Health Physician Partners—are working to change health care for the better. We're making breakthroughs in medicine at the Feinstein Institutes for Medical Research. We're training the next generation of medical professionals at the visionary Donald and Barbara Zucker School of Medicine at Hofstra/Northwell and the Hofstra Northwell School of Nursing and Physician Assistant Studies. For information on our more than 100 medical specialties, visit Northwell.edu and follow us @NorthwellHealth on Facebook, Twitter, Instagram, and LinkedIn.

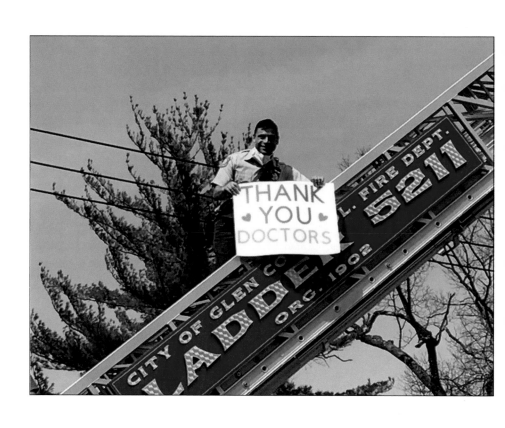

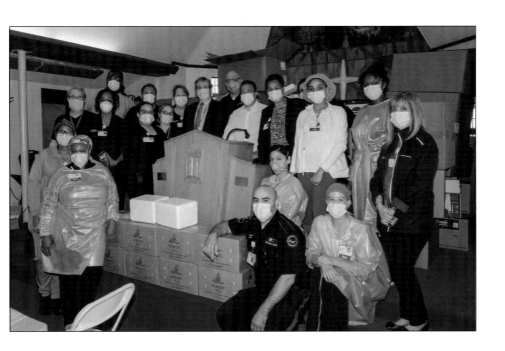

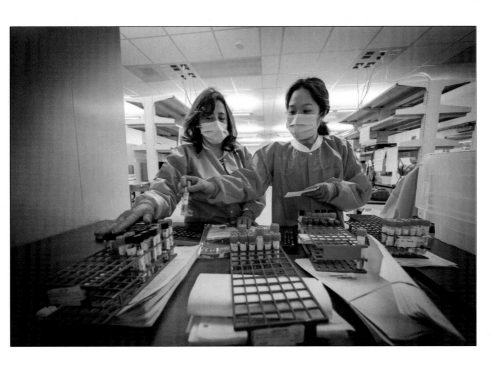

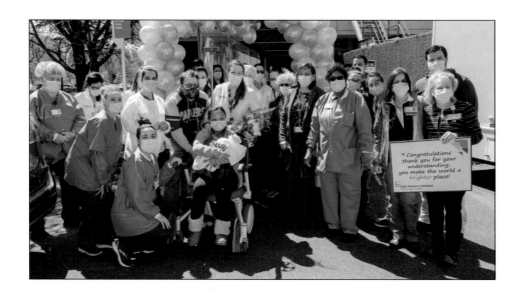

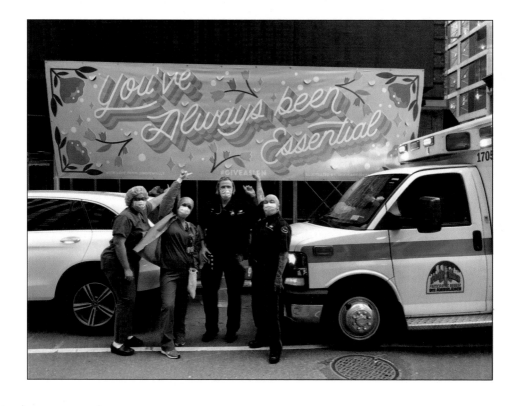

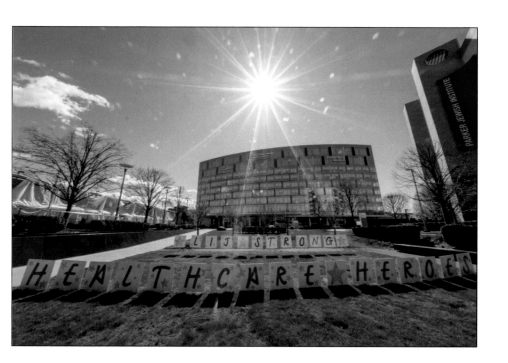

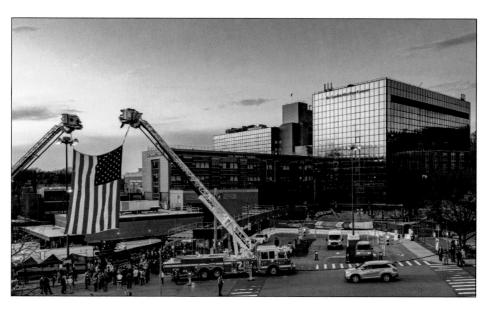

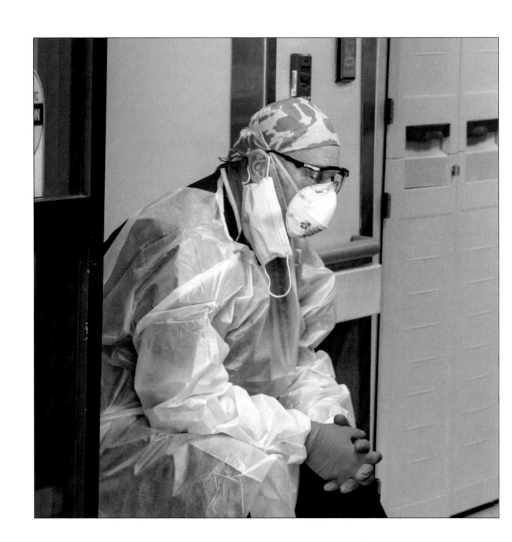

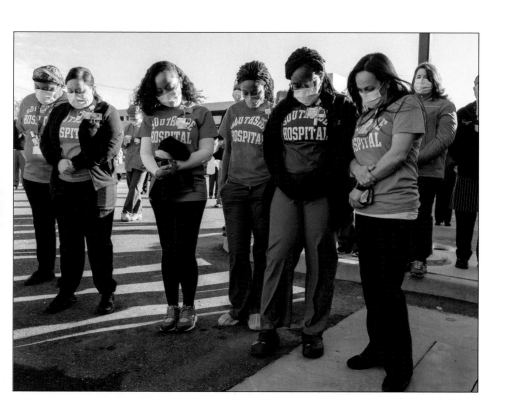

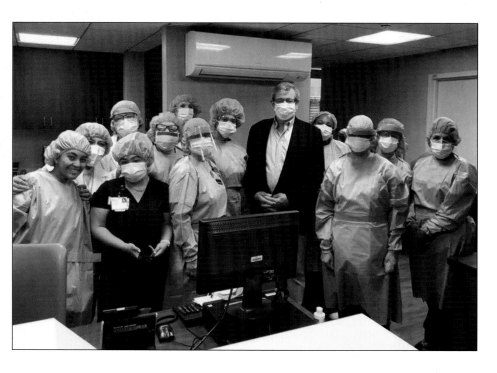

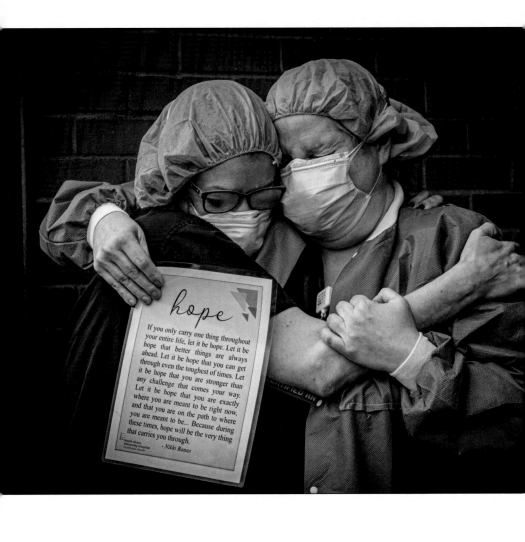

series of suppliers from around the world, including stepped-up domestic production. American-made items will be far more expensive than Chinese-made goods, but the necessity for US based manufacturing could not be clearer.

But in January and February, McCready and Drummond were not yet thinking about creating a supply chain less reliant on China. They were focused on getting the PPE and other equipment that the clinical and support teams at Northwell would need. And as the weeks passed, it became clear to McCready that with the virus headed to New York, the need could be enormous. She bought gowns, face shields, and procedural masks by the millions. She purchased five times as many N95 masks as she normally ordered—more than she had ever ordered at one time. These were made by 3M in the United Kingdom, but she was concerned that the material supply line from China to the United Kingdom could be disrupted.

One evening, while at home with her mother watching television, there was news from China about the coronavirus and how the spread was forcing Chinese authorities to lock down certain areas, including Wuhan. A scene came on the news of a gray-haired woman from China, out in public, a drone hovering above her and a voice telling her to go home and remain isolated. "And I said to my mother, 'That could never happen here, right?'" McCready recalled.

To which her mother replied, "The world is very small, Phyllis.'"

And McCready said, "You're right. It could happen here!"

* * *

The news out of Italy was terrifying. McCready and Donna Drummond saw and read about frontline staff dying in some cases due to lack of protective gear. At the same time, aware of the amount of travel between New York and various Italian cities, it was clear that the virus was on its way. At Northwell we had a good base of supplies to begin with and that base was supplemented significantly by the orders the team had put in during the week of January 17. But now, in late February, as Italy was about to be inundated, the push was on to buy even more. By this point, however, every hospital in the country was in the market for more

PPE and ventilators. We were competing with every major health system and every state government, as well as the federal government. It was madness.

Drummond said that one of Northwell's greatest advantages during the worldwide hunt for more PPE and other supplies was Phyllis McCready's decades of experience and the hundreds of relationships with vendors she had developed through the years. "Phyllis has done an incredible job," Drummond said. "Relationships with vendors can be transactional and adversarial, but she's always been very fair. They always respect her. They respect her knowledge. They respect her intelligence, that she knows their product. These direct relationships are incredibly beneficial in times of emergency. The vendors know us, know we will pay them, and are anxious to meet our needs. Throughout this event, our vendors have been working incredibly hard to get to us what they can. For example, 3M has never stopped delivering nor raised their prices for N95 masks. Unfortunately, they haven't been able to satisfy the increased demand. Cardinal and Dukal have also been great partners."

As the marketplace of available equipment contracted, McCready found that the very large volumes she was accustomed to purchasing were unavailable. She and the team began placing multiple orders for smaller lots, taking whatever they could get. In normal times, she might buy a half million or a million masks, for example. Now she was finding that she had to do much smaller orders. Swabs, used for taking a culture from a patient's nasal passage, were running low, and McCready put in orders for three thousand, then five thousand. She got 2,500. On top of that, she was finding that shipments took longer than usual. Part of the issue was that suppliers were doing their best to get PPE to where it was most urgently needed, which at that time was Europe. When we at Northwell place a purchase order, the process of filling and shipping that order begins overseas. McCready told the team to continue placing orders even if they had open, unfilled orders for the same material. She was counting on the rule that as long as she had open orders, things had to ship.

The main vendors, Cardinal and 3M, were inundated with demands for supplies and equipment from across the world, but they were open with our teams and said honestly what they could and could not do.

And that is what we needed—transparency. If they assured us something was in the pipeline and on its way, it was true. Sometimes delivery dates shifted and were delayed, but we eventually got our orders filled.

* * *

In March the data was telling McCready and Drummond that usage of gowns, masks, and other equipment was starting to climb. This was the perfect storm McCready worried about: increased demand, reduced supply. "I knew we were going to have a problem," she recalled. As the patient census climbed so, too, did the staff's need for PPE. At one point in March the need for isolation gowns, for example, rose from an average of about 8,500 per day to more than fifty-five thousand per day. We went from using about 18,600 N95 masks a month to using about eight thousand per day—225,000 per month. This skyrocketing usage put

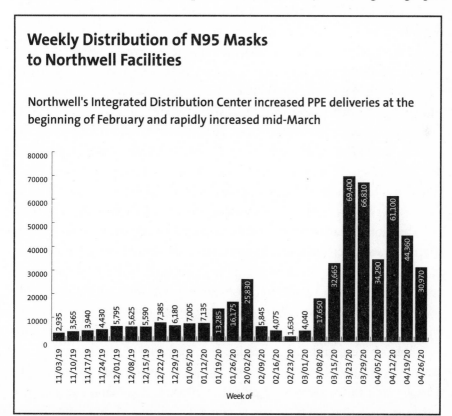

Weekly Distribution of N95 Masks to Northwell Facilities

Northwell's Integrated Distribution Center increased PPE deliveries at the beginning of February and rapidly increased mid-March

Week of

tremendous pressure on Drummond, McCready, and their team to find new sources for N95 masks. Historically, these masks were worn by clinicians in the presence of confirmed pulmonary/laryngeal tuberculosis, measles, and chicken pox. At some facilities, staff would use the mask once and discard it; at others they'd only discard it at the end of the shift. The CDC's recommendation was that the mask be used throughout a full shift and then discarded. With the rapidly increasing number of COVID patients, however, the ability to purchase N95s became more of a challenge, and the CDC issued a ruling allowing the use of the masks past the manufacturer's designated shelf life date. It also exempted users from conducting a fit test. Employees were asked to use the mask for a full shift unless it got wet or otherwise compromised. The goal was to emphasize the need to extend and reuse N95s to enable ongoing availability for employees treating COVID-positive patients. Reuse of these masks became standard practice during the crisis.

Drummond, McCready, and their colleagues called upon every vendor they could find to try and buy more. "We continued to receive the masks from 3M although not in the volume we were asking for," said McCready. "And then word came from 3M that they could not deliver any more to us." One alternative was to order additional procedural masks, the thinner masks that prevent the wearer from spreading germs but do not protect the wearer from an airborne virus. A delivery of ten million procedural masks arrived in March, but there was a slight issue: The masks were being held at JFK and would not be released by the Port Authority. Fortunately, the appropriate officials found a way to enlist the support of the managers at JFK and the Teamsters to release the shipment.

The global marketplace for PPE and other equipment was a chaotic space. We were getting scores of cold calls from vendors we'd never heard of who claimed they had access to large supplies of PPE. We received countless calls from people and companies claiming to have large supplies of N95 masks, as well as gowns and even ventilators. The problem with nearly every one of them was lack of transparency. They might send a sample so we could judge quality, but we had no guarantee that the sample represented the quality of the full shipment; or even if there would actually be a full shipment. Typically, with these cold calls, the contract would require that we place the payment—millions of dollars—into an escrow account. The stipulation was that when we signed the contract, the funds would be released to the seller from the account. But this left us with no guarantee of getting quality goods or any goods at all. There were countless leads where somebody knew somebody whose friend had access to a large supply. None of these deals worked out. And even when we did receive much-needed ventilators from New York State, many arrived without parts needed to make them functional. At one point our staff members went to hardware stores to purchase garden hoses which they cut up and attached so vents would work. At another point, through a highly reliable company, we placed an order for one million N95s. Instead of the old price of less than a dollar per mask, the new asking price was more than seven dollars. The deal was on, or so it seemed. But the shipment was in Mexico where the government placed an additional tax on the masks, driving the cost up over ten dollars each. In the end, the Mexican government would not permit the masks to be shipped out of the country. Governor Cuomo made sure the state government filled in some of the gaps with the N95s, and private donors contributed masks as well, including PwC and Goldman Sachs. There were some supplies from China for which the shipping cost exceeded the price of the goods themselves. This was true when we needed a rush order and had the goods flown to JFK via air freight rather than shipped across the ocean and then trucked to New York.

In New York State, early projections suggested that ventilators might well be in short supply at the peak of the pandemic. We purchased four hundred new vents and although we did not end up receiving all of them, we always had sufficient quantities, in large measure because of our system's ability to move equipment rapidly to wherever it was needed among our twenty-three hospitals. The state pitched in with two hundred and provided additional PPE, as well.

We were helped during the crisis by the generosity of private donors. When the pandemic struck we were in the thick of a multiyear effort to raise a billion dollars in private gifts, but when the virus was coming our way we shifted gears virtually overnight to try and raise funds to support our efforts throughout the crisis. "We had been talking to the communities (we served) about our cancer programs and about resources and buildings," said Brian Lally, chief development officer, "and we just pulled the plug on all of it, and then went all in on communicating about what we're doing on the COVID side. And we got an outpouring of support from the broader communities, both at our hospitals and at the system level."

Many people made generous gifts hoping it would help us secure the PPE and equipment we needed. Our communities knew that we would be taking a massive financial hit, and they wanted to do what they could to soften the blow. We also received many in-kind donations of N95 masks and ventilators—more than a million items in all! Other offerings from the communities we serve were smaller, more discreet, but more meaningful than anything else: Individuals and families bought lunches and dinners and delivered them to our hospitals. We learned throughout that people were eager to help, and they would ask us what they could do in various ways large and small. This all helped financially, but it also boosted morale. When our teams know that the communities are with us, that they will support us through this, it is truly uplifting.

Some of the most meaningful gifts came from members of our board of trustees, the volunteer leaders who play a crucial role in guiding this organization forward. One hundred percent of board members made gifts and went out and raised additional money.

* * *

As we approached the peak, concern grew throughout the greater New York area about the possibility of not having enough ventilators for all the patients needing one. This was the stuff of our worst nightmares. Yes, we had a policy based on rigorous ethical, clinical, and legal analysis that would guide us in making a decision: Two patients, one ventilator—who gets it? While we had the policy, we certainly never wanted to use it and, fortunately, we never did. While we worked our sources to find ventilators, we also went to work trying to figure out whether there might be alternatives in an emergency. Some very clever scientists and engineers in our system came up with a viable alternative. BiPAP machines are commonly used among people with sleep apnea to provide positive airway pressure (PAP) that helps them maintain a consistent breathing pattern at night. The machines are also commonly used with patients suffering from congestive heart failure or from chronic inflammatory lung disease

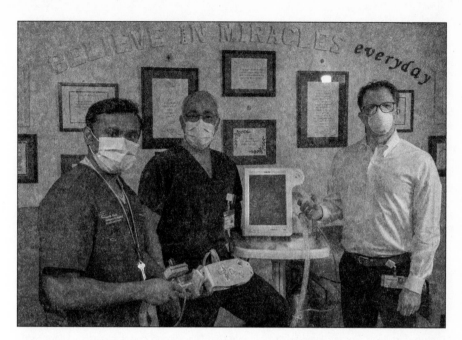

Pictured is the team that made the conversion of BiPAP machines possible.

such as chronic obstructive pulmonary disease (COPD). In other words, like ventilators, these machines help patients breathe.

Dr. Hugh Cassiere, medical director for respiratory therapy services, and Stanley John, director of respiratory therapy at North Shore University Hospital, developed a method to convert a BiPAP into a pressure-controlled ventilator that could be used on patients with COVID-19 (or any other patients for that matter). But there was a catch: Their invention would not

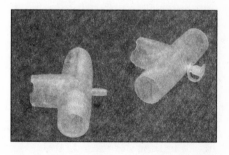

This is an example of the 3D-printed pieces used to convert BiPAP machines to ventilators.

work without an essential part—a small, plastic, T-piece adapter.

And these were in short supply—so short that we were unable to get any. Enter Todd Goldstein, PhD, director of 3D design and innovation at Northwell. The three men collaborated to come up with a way to design a 3D-printed T-piece. They tested it successfully and set to producing dozens of the 3D-printed pieces so that they could convert BiPAP

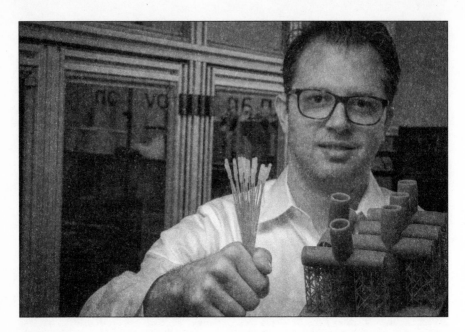

Pictured is Todd Goldstein who led the team that 3D-printed nasal swabs for diagnostic testing.

machines when the patient load was heaviest. In another bit of innovative magic, our team in collaboration with the University of South Florida and Formlabs, a 3D printing company, produced 3D-printed nasal swabs needed to test patients for the virus, swabs which were at that point in woefully short supply throughout the country.

* * *

One of the lessons Phyllis McCready takes from the COVID-19 experience is that she intends to be better prepared in understanding where everything is coming from. "I don't just want to know where the manufacturing plants are making the products; I want to know the origin of the raw materials and the full path to completion of the product," she said. The problem with ventilators, for example, was not that companies wouldn't ramp up their production. Rather, they did not have the parts they needed in order to ramp up their production, because those parts were coming from China.

Donna Drummond observes that, in the future, prices for some items will rise because within our system we will insist upon buying some supplies manufactured in America. In fact, while the crisis was still going on in May, we were exploring the possibility of purchasing a PPE manufacturing company located in the United States so that we and others will have a steady supply of domestically made equipment and supplies in the future. And a major improvement Drummond envisions is an investment in automation to update our supply-chain systems "so that we have the information that we need more readily available to manage our supplies. We have to become more like Walmart in terms of automation—to know where the equipment is and who is using it at any given moment. Our goal needs to be a better understanding of the cost of care, including supplies, as well as the ability to better track them. This goes beyond emergency preparedness."

Our supply team scoured the world for masks and other protective equipment, for ventilators, for swabs, for everything that every other major health system in the world was competing for, and they came up with the products to protect our staff and care for our patients. But this entire process needs a massive overhaul at the national and even international level. In the crisis we were required to pay seven dollars—or even ten dollars—for fifty-cent masks. We were asked to pay ten times the normal rate to hire temporary nurses. Even in cases where our teams were able to find the needed product, we weren't always certain—until it actually arrived—that it met our quality standards. As many others have noted, the idea that our organization, other health-care systems, our nation, and the world rely upon China almost exclusively for the manufacture of these crucial items is a dangerous gamble. Domestic production of essential supplies is a matter of national security in the future.

Toward that end, during the pandemic in April our health system joined a new IBM block chain network called Rapid Supplier Connect. McCready was very familiar with the vendors we traditionally worked with, but looking for and vetting new vendors was a complicated and time-consuming task. The IBM system was established specifically to help organizations connect quickly with new suppliers during the pandemic and beyond. The IBM technology made finding matches between buyers and sellers of particular equipment and supplies much faster.

CHAPTER SIX

Clinical Decision-Making in a Pandemic

Lessons

- A structured clinical advisory team is one of the more important components of emergency management in a crisis.
- The clinical advisory team's ability to continuously issue alerts, policies, best practice guidelines, and clarifications on clinical policy is an absolute key to success.
- Frequent communication (often daily) about what exactly is going on clinically and what lies ahead enhances staff confidence and treatment methodologies, and also reduces staff anxiety and fear.
- Close cooperation between clinical and operational leaders promotes efficient implementation.
- Enhancing testing capabilities must become a priority.

In a matter of days, we transformed our system into a massive series of specialty hospitals and ambulatory facilities caring for nearly fifty thousand patients with COVID-19. It is impossible to describe how surreal this experience was. As Dr. McGinn put it during the crisis: "It does seem unreal even when you're in the middle of it. You're like, 'This can't really be happening, right?'"

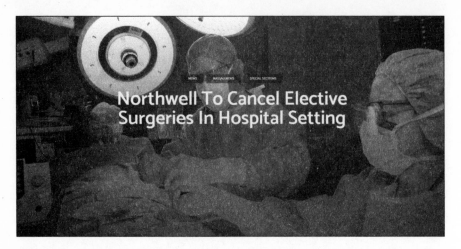

One of the most significant early decisions was to cancel all elective surgeries. Source: *Long Island Weekly*

A central capability within our incident command structure comes from our clinical advisory group, a team led by Dr. Mark Jarrett that also includes Drs. John D'Angelo, Annabella Salvador-Kelly, Thomas McGinn, Dwayne Breining, and Bruce Farber, as well as Donna Armellino, vice president of infection prevention. This team provided medical guidance to the incident commanders, who were overseeing the entire emergency operation. Given that little was known about the coronavirus that meant updating clinical practice guidelines daily and sometimes even more frequently as we accumulated information and experience. The physicians played a central role in every decision, ranging from whether to halt elective surgery to our no-visitor policy to who should be placed on a ventilator and when. Without the clinical group, the incident commanders would be unable to function.

The advisory group faced multiple clinical challenges during the pandemic, not the least of which was the transformation to a patient mix that was overwhelmingly COVID. And with the intensity of the work, it often felt as though we were doing nothing but COVID. (We did continue providing care for patients with heart disease, cancer, and the like. Cancer patients who needed radiation and chemotherapy got it as needed. The OB department continued to deliver babies.) Our physicians on the emergency operations team did what they had long planned to do: study the reality, weigh the evidence, review the data, and make evidence-based decisions about care. But there was a problem: Neither they nor any other medical professionals in the world knew much of anything about the coronavirus. Certainly, the news out of China had not been particularly clarifying. Our doctors knew that the disease caused acute respiratory distress that was fatal in some cases, but little else. "We heard things from China, but their data was not clear," said Jarrett. "All of their reports in the literature were more about, 'Five cases were treated this way. Ten cases were treated this way.' But no real, large studies."

Ideally, we wanted to standardize best practice treatments across the system for the simple reason that studies have shown that standardized care for certain conditions improves both outcomes and safety. The advisory group worked together to standardize care and provide clinical guidelines for frontline clinicians based on what they knew about respiratory care and what little data they had. Organizations such as the Joint Commission, the Institute for Healthcare Improvement, and the New York State Department of Health have promoted the establishment of standardization when a clear best practice has been demonstrated by evidence. But doctors tend to be independent thinkers and standardizing care has been difficult to accomplish. The pandemic was one of those clarifying events that actually helped us focus on a few best practices and seek to standardize them throughout our system.

Our physician clinical group leaders developed scores of protocols to guide frontline staff in making consistent decisions about treatments. For example, our doctors confirmed through early observations that a significant percentage of patients with COVID were suffering from blood clots. We established guidelines for which patients should be given anti-coagulant medication and when they should get it. In addition, the treatment guidelines provided doctors with a way of navigating situations in which patients that had not been admitted but were recovering at home should receive anti-coagulants. Another example involved what medicine generally to give to patients. In May, the FDA approved the antiviral agent Remdesivir for use in patients with the virus. The problem was that Remdesivir was in relatively short supply. So our physician leaders defined a calculus guiding doctors on which patients would benefit most from it and which patients would likely not benefit. Based on the science involved, we established a tier system that prioritized patients whose conditions made them most likely to benefit from the drug.

The most sobering policy involved the question of life-sustaining treatments in a crisis situation. Our policy, issued during the height of the crisis, "is a theoretical construct for a *what if* situation we hope never occurs," said Dr. David Battinelli. And the situation we hope never occurs is the rationing of care based on limited availability of medicines or technology. In the case of the coronavirus, the policy we issued was based on a theoretical case in which we would find ourselves with an insufficient number of ventilators for all the patients needing those machines. We were not running out of ventilators and, in fact, at no time did we experience a ventilator shortage. But early on that was a concern, and thus our ethical committee in concert with clinicians developed a policy to provide guidance should the situation occur. The policy, said Battinelli, "doesn't tell you what to do. It makes sure that you look at the problem from an ethical viewpoint and consider who will benefit the most." One consideration in the ethical equation of deciding who gets a ventilator and who does not, for example, might be the fact that no patient over the age of eighty-five has survived the virus on a ventilator. That said, we had no rules based on age or any other demographic indicator. Our policy was leaked to the press, which was fine with us because we had a perfectly reasonable explanation for it, which one of us (Michael Dowling) articulated when he was interviewed on *Face the Nation*: "You have to have a policy prepared well in advance. I don't think we will ever get to that point, but it would be foolish to wait until you have a disaster and then try to develop the policy . . . during that situation. So this is all preparation. It's just the draft. It's not happening. We hope it never happens. But if it does, we are prepared."

We established standards for employees, requiring any staff member exposed to the virus to quarantine for fourteen days, but even that became problematic when hundreds of staff members were home quarantined and we faced staffing shortages. Revised CDC guidance allowed the person exposed to continue working if he or she showed no symptoms. An early standard practice, as mentioned in chapter 2, required all employees to wear masks to protect themselves and to reduce the spread to patients and other workers. This mandate came before any other health system in the state instituted a mandatory mask policy and even before the CDC issued a similar guideline. Our data later showed that getting masks on

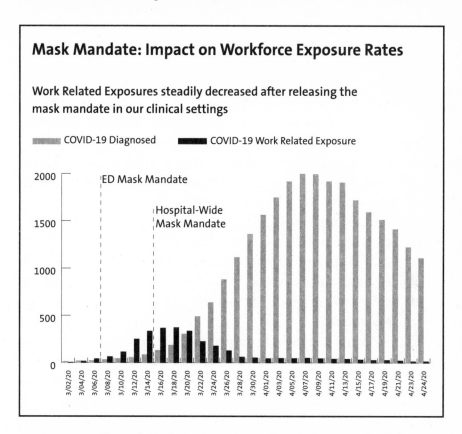

Mask Mandate: Impact on Workforce Exposure Rates

Work Related Exposures steadily decreased after releasing the mask mandate in our clinical settings

COVID-19 Diagnosed   COVID-19 Work Related Exposure

employees at that relatively early point reduced the spread of the virus among staff. "We did that because we felt that would offer more protection not only for the staff but for other patients," said Dr. John D'Angelo, "and in retrospect, that was a very good decision because of the fact that we didn't have a lot of testing in the beginning, and there were people who had been admitted for what we thought were non-COVID lung problems or other problems. When we got testing ramped up six, seven days later it turned out they did have COVID."

* * *

We established a standard process for evaluating patients presenting in our emergency departments, starting with an assessment: What suggested that this patient might be COVID positive? Initially, patients who had recently traveled to China, Italy, or Iran were likely candidates. Patients with fever, cough, and difficulty breathing were also candidates.

For most patients, especially young healthy people, the best course of action was to ride out the disease at home. Tens of thousands came to our urgent care centers, and most of these patients were also able to recover at home. Several thousand that we examined in our EDs were sick but nonetheless able to manage at home, although a small percentage of these patients returned much sicker and were admitted.

At a higher acuity level were patients presenting in our EDs with respiratory distress. Any patient not oxygenating well and with labored breathing was admitted. We learned over time that symptoms varied. Some patients experienced generalized body pain, fatigue, persistent cough, stomach pain, diarrhea, or headache. But the key factors in identifying a COVID patient centered on oxygen levels and difficulty breathing. These people were admitted to our hospitals through the ED and moved to the units as quickly as possible so that our EDs would not become overwhelmed.

One of the many problems throughout the pandemic was the question of how exactly to treat patients once they were up on the unit. The unknown nature of the virus made creating treatment protocols challenging. "There's a lot of stuff out in the press where people say, 'oh this is great' and some of it may be, but we really don't know," said Jarrett. "And you can't give all the medicines because some conflict with others. So we have to figure out based on the studies we're doing what are the best therapies."

Every patient that showed up in our ED who required admission was tested for the virus, given a chest X-ray, and, in most cases, put on oxygen. The progression of the disease was different for different patients. Some were stable for a couple of days, then crashed. Others collapsed in the ED having gone from a normal blood oxygen saturation in the 95 to 100 percent range down to 75 or 80 percent within hours. There were some patients who, while awaiting test results, would experience extreme pulmonary problems. In general, we followed the Acute Respiratory Distress Syndrome Net protocol (ARDSnet), a NIH agreed-upon protocol for acute lung injury.

The differences in symptoms and the rate and manner of disease progression made it hard to know exactly how to treat COVID patients. The lack of clarity was evident in a late March memorandum from physician leaders to doctors throughout our system:

The clinical advisory team is revising our clinical protocols on a daily basis as we gather information shared by practitioners from around the world. We remain committed to proceed based on available evidence, best common practice, and clinical judgment, and weighing known risks and benefits . . . Despite all best efforts and attempts at consensus of optimal treatment strategies, the virus pathogenesis and mechanisms are still largely undefined, and we continue to have enormous challenges for patients suffering and dying. It is critical that we maintain an approach based on science and evidence and continue with clinical trials. Our objective, stringent, and not anecdotal results are critical as we move forward ourselves, and as we provide data for the rest of the country. We are the front line and bear exceptional responsibility and burdens.

That said, it is understandable additional therapies (e.g. high dose steroids, off label medications including interleukin inhibitors and anti-viral therapies, and others), although unproven, will be entertained and advocated by both well-intentioned clinicians and concerned families. Based on the guidance from the Clinical Operations and COVID-19 Research Committee, we are in agreement that decisions regarding such therapies will be the responsibility of the clinicians and the local medical leadership at each institution and based on individual patient needs.

In the early stages of the pandemic, the reality, said Dr. Lawrence Smith, was:

that we knew literally nothing about it. The things that the disease did were continuous surprises. We also didn't know the level of contagion. Certainly, when people got on a ventilator early on that was really a sign that they were very likely to not get out of the hospital alive. The demand to try *anything* was enormous, regardless of whether there was a shred of proof that anything worked. And then, each time we got something new in or learned something new, we changed protocol. Each time another hospital reported, *hey this worked* or *this doesn't work* we changed the protocol because nobody knew anything about what really should be done to these patients. I think we created a level of "the protocol of the day," never mind the week, that was disconcerting to the staff and hard to remember. It was hard to remember *just exactly what am I supposed to do today that's different from what I did yesterday?*

Establishing standard best practices for treating COVID patients was difficult, because the disease was brand new and we kept learning as we went along. Thus, our standard work recommendations changed frequently. Our standard practice, particularly for patients who deteriorated to the point where they required intubation, included specific vent settings, types of sedation used, and whether—and when—to perform a tracheotomy. We also turned patients over onto their stomachs ("proning") to improve lung function. "We had a lot of staff who really had never taken care of patients on ventilators before who were now helping," said Jarrett. "Therefore, by having a standard protocol, it made it easier for them to follow treatment based on evidence that was present at the time." The drug protocols were a scramble because there were so many different indications early on of what might work and what wasn't working. That was frustrating for all the doctors involved. At various times we tried hydroxychloroquine or Zithromax. Nothing worked.

The variable nature of the disease seemed to get more rather than less confounding as the contagion spread. Early on, conventional wisdom was that the very old and the severely immune-compromised were at greatest risk of fatal illness, but "we had older people who came in and were sick for five or six days in the hospital and then they'd be able to go home," said Jarrett. "We also had relatively young people, in their forties or fifties, who came into the emergency room, the first two days were fine, and then on day three all of a sudden their oxygen level dropped to very low levels, and they wound up needing to be in the ICU and ventilated." There was no predictability to how any given patient would react. But the unexpected rapid deterioration of otherwise healthy people was alarming. It was not something with which we were accustomed to dealing in our hospitals, where it is highly unusual for a generally healthy person to come in and crash a day later.

Surge planning anticipated that sick patients would need a respirator for a standard length of time—four or five days was about the norm in the pre-COVID world. But doctors were discovering that COVID patients survived who were ventilated for as long as three or four *weeks*. "We didn't know that would happen with this virus," said Jarrett. "We didn't know that patients would be on two to four weeks." Frontline physicians, nurses, physician assistants, nurse practitioners, and respiratory therapists saw an unpredictable mix of patients for whom the severity of illness changed over time. Many patients required levels of oxygen that we had never seen before.

But not all was doom and gloom. Over the course of the onslaught, we learned a tremendous amount about caring for the sickest patients. We got a better sense of the disease with each passing day and that taught us to place patients on ventilators at certain times and no earlier; it taught us to set ventilator oxygen levels in certain ranges depending upon the patient's condition. These and other lessons caused the survival rate of our patients on ventilators to improve from 20 percent early on to approximately 40 percent later in the crisis. Dr. Lawrence Smith said that success was a result of "fanatically good critical care; that improvement did not come from any specific drug. It came from understanding the rhythm of when these people were going to get bad so that you could intervene a little earlier, and then just fanatically good critical care at a level that we have never done for any other disease."

What does that care look like in practical terms? Smith continued:

> The way the ventilator was used, the positioning of the patients, the way you used pressure agents to support blood pressure, anticipating the kidney failure; it was just really, really good critical care medicine with no room for error and no room for missing what was going to happen or for the clues that were being found in the patient. We just got better and better and better at that. Part of it was understanding the rhythm of this disease, which is unlike any disease that any of us have ever treated before. And so, slowly but surely, learning. Plus, we

had a lot of docs in those critical care units that weren't critical care docs because we didn't have enough critical care docs
for [the] two thousand more ICU beds that we created. So,
you had to have critical care leaders telling people who didn't
usually even do this stuff how to do it right, but we got much,
much better at it.

By early May we had discharged more than ten thousand COVID
patients from our hospitals; people who had been very sick yet had survived. Still, our work was not done when they went home. We conducted
virtual follow-up visits and we sent many patients home with pulse oxim-
eters to measure blood oxygen level. Many other patients went home
with anticoagulation medicine to prevent blood clots. Many patients
who have spent extended periods of time on ventilators emerge from the
hospital in a dramatically weakened condition and thus require physical
therapy, which is done virtually. Thus, even after patients survived and
were discharged, there was still more work to do to care for them at
home. Fortunately, we have an extensive home care network that kicked
into gear and made thousands of virtual home visits to care for patients.

* * *

For Dr. Jarrett, there were a number of lessons from the experience. "You
really do need an incident command system because there are so many
moving parts that you must have it organized in that fashion," he said.
He also cited the value of standardization:

> The use of clinical groups to develop algorithms and pathways
> and standards was critical because otherwise we had one hos-
> pital doing one thing, one hospital doing another. Sometimes
> there's more than one way to do something. It's not that one
> is necessarily better than the other. There are controversies in
> medicine, but where it made a big impact is: We were moving
> staff around all over the place because of the load balancing
> and things we were doing, and you don't want staff being at one
> hospital doing it one way and then going to another hospital

and everybody's doing it another way. That becomes dangerous, so that's why we needed to really standardize things with
obvious exceptions for particular clinical situations.

Another lesson is that frequent communication about exactly what is
going on, and what may be coming down the road, helps reduce staff
anxiety and fear. And within that lesson is another: "As much as you
think you can predict how much stress this produces for the staff you'll
really underestimate it, because unlike other situations that we've all gone
through, this is a very long event," said Jarrett. "It's an event that unfortunately is associated with a lot of death and much more than people
are used to, which is a huge stress. It becomes a super-stressful situation,
which, although we anticipated it, you don't recognize what impact this
is having on your staff until it's going on for four or five weeks."

No one had seen death rates this high. Throughout our system, doctors and nurses were having exceptionally difficult end-of-life conversations
with families whose loved ones were rapidly deteriorating on ventilators.
These were the types of conversations that typically would be held pri-
vately and in person. In normal times, families are present and can see
firsthand how bad a patient's condition is. But in the time of COVID,
end-of-life conversations were held at the bedside, where the patient was
generally unaware of what was going on. In many cases our doctors and
nurses would connect with the family at home via FaceTime. This enabled
loved ones to see how badly the patient had deteriorated and that gave
them a better sense of what was to come.

While our planning efforts worked well overall, one thing we had
not and maybe could not have planned for was the depth of emotional
strain on our staff. "We knew, but we didn't understand, the unbelievable
impact of caring for people who became living corpses," said Dr. Smith.

They were on ventilators, stacked bed-to-bed in ICUs, para-
lyzed, sedated, never moved a muscle, never blinked, and had
no relatives there to advocate for them. It became like a living
morgue. The only thing that changed was when they died,
and when they died that was a failure, a failure of staff and
everybody else. That was an unbelievably stressful situation to

put people in day after day, without any of the humanness, the rewards of interacting with the patient and the patient smiling at you and thanking you. Even somebody giving you a hard time because you're not taking good care of their relative. There just was nobody around. It was dead silent.

So much illness and death. A grim message sent to the clinical staff on May 1 reported that:

> [A] New York—Presbyterian physician who tragically committed suicide this week is a sobering reminder of the physical, mental, and emotional toll that the COVID-19 pandemic is having on caregivers, including physicians. Dr. Lorna Breen completed her residency training at Northwell approximately fifteen years ago, which hits even closer to home for those who may have known her.
>
> As physicians, you are used to responding to tragedies and crises. And while we are seeing signs of hope amidst the grave challenge you've faced, the scale and intensity of the pandemic, in addition to individual concerns about getting sick and infecting colleagues and family members, has enhanced the need to care for our caregivers.

The message then reminded doctors of the help available to them via a number of emotional guidance and support programs.

* * *

The most frustrating aspect of the crisis from a clinical perspective involved testing for the virus—or, more accurately, the inability to test on a broad basis. The word early on that came to Dr. Dwayne Breining, the head of the Northwell laboratory, was that the FDA was taking a position that no tests from labs like ours would be approved because the CDC was setting up testing for the entire nation. This meant that the major manufacturers of medical tests were barred from developing and selling their own tests. When the CDC did release its test, it proved to be defective. This is a classic example of failing to prepare for a crisis. The virus was out there and it was coming to America—that was clear. Why wouldn't we as a nation welcome large testing companies with excellent track records on other types of tests to market tens of millions of tests throughout the country? "I have no idea what the rationale for that was," said Breining. "It makes no reasonable sense whatsoever in terms of responding to the crisis. There was a lot of grumbling in the professional laboratory community in the US." An online petition was signed by thousands of lab professionals with the message that, as Breining described it, "this restriction is unnecessarily delaying what is a true patient care need. And, based on that, I think the FDA reversed course and then opened up this emergency use authorization pathway to allow laboratories to set up testing in their laboratories and develop their own tests, which also opened the door to the manufacturers at that time."

In New York, we went to work on a test and collaborated on that effort with the team at the New York State lab that specializes in analysis and investigations related to threats to public health, and with whom we have a strong relationship. Governor Cuomo was instrumental in speeding up the process so that we could begin working on developing what is known as a PCR test, which determines whether a person is infected with the virus. We shared testing material and data with the state lab team and we were able to develop a test in our lab on March 8. The problem was that because it was a purely manual test, we could not produce nearly the quantity needed to test our patients. "It's not an automated test at all," Breining said, "so it requires basically some of my most highly skilled techs in the laboratory to run it, and basically occupies them for the whole time that they're running it . . . and even then the most that could be produced were about seventy-five to eighty tests a day." Soon thereafter we were able to improve with a semi-automated test and then, finally in April, a fully automated test that enabled us to test two thousand people per day. It was progress, but "it was still frustrating. At every step of the way you still feel frustrated because you know you're only hitting about one-tenth of what you would like your target to be."

By May, we were able to conduct serology tests that revealed whether or not a person has had the infection and whether that person has developed antibodies to the virus. There is not yet certainty about whether

patients who have been infected with the virus are immune from rein-
fection, but the generally accepted medical view is that it is more likely
than not.

We also worked to make these tests more widely available to help
communities determine the prevalence of the virus. We were able to set
up dozens of testing centers for our own employees as well as for first
responders, including police and firefighters, state police, employees of
the corrections department, and the MTA. At the request of Governor
Cuomo, we sent out teams into forty churches in Black, Latino, and
other communities where the population was disproportionately harmed
by COVID. Employee testing confirmed that the steps we had taken
to protect our employees had worked well. By late spring, one of our
physicians, Dr. James Crawford, was leading a consortium of all laboratories in New York in an ongoing process of validating various tests and
determining which labs had significant testing capacity. Eventually, our
lab developed the capacity to conduct more than seven thousand PCR
tests per day and in excess of twenty-five thousand serology tests per day.

* * *

One of the many clinical concerns facing our physician leaders—despite
all the beds we'd created across the system, and the streamlining of
patient transfers from overstretched facilities—was the need for additional capacity outside our system. Here is where the Javits Center and
USNS *Comfort* were helpful in making a combined total of two thousand beds available. As our doctors and nurses were struggling to keep
up with growing numbers, Governor Cuomo pressed the federal government for help. The Navy dispatched the *Comfort,* which docked in New
York Harbor on March 30, and at the same time the National Guard and
Army Corps of Engineers transformed the Javits Center into a makeshift
hospital. That was the initial good news. Then came the bad news. The
problem was that both of these temporary facilities were supposed to be
reserved for patients with medical conditions other than COVID, when
the reality at the front lines was that all over the region we were inundated
with almost nothing but COVID. On top of that was confusion at the
Javits Center about which patients could be admitted there. Eventually,

state officials asked our team at Northwell to step in and help manage the situation. It was a tough challenge. Hospitals throughout the region were pushed to maximum capacity and beyond. Having a safety valve of more than a thousand beds at the Javits Center could be a lifeline. Yet as enticing as the Javits capacity was, none of the health systems were having any luck getting patients admitted there. Mark Solazzo knew that the Javits pipeline had to be opened up, and on the morning of April 3, a Friday, he called Rita Mercieca, a senior vice president at Northwell, and asked her to visit the Javits Center that afternoon to meet with state officials. She did so, and by 7:00 a.m. the next morning Mercieca was coordinating efforts to get patients into Javits.

Eligibility guidelines for patients to be admitted to the Javits Center were far too restrictive, and there was a tangled bureaucratic process to fight through in order to get a patient admitted. "Hospitals were trying to get patients in, and it would take up to two to three hours to get one patient accepted," said Mercieca. "They were giving up. These doctors were tired, and they were being asked to spend three hours on the phone and then do clerical stuff and just ridiculous things that were making it so hard to get a patient in that they were just giving up."

An important moment came when all of the chief medical officers from organizations involved with Javits—the Navy, the state, the New York City Department of Health, the Army, and the National Guard—gathered together and visited Lenox Hill Hospital in Manhattan, part of the Northwell system. Our doctors at Lenox Hill had fresh experience with the disease and they explained that patients sick with COVID who were beginning their recovery would be safe to move to Javits. After the Lenox Hill meeting, the various chief medical officers put their heads together and agreed on a set of criteria for patients who would be admitted to Javits, including COVID-positive patients. Establishing the criteria for admission was key, for it enabled Mercieca and her colleagues to scan data and identify patients fitting the criteria. Mercieca's plan from the start was to go out to crowded hospitals, identify patients who fit the criteria, and *pull* them into Javits. Until then, physicians seeking to move a patient to Javits had to *push* the patient in through a bureaucratic maze. It wasn't working. Instead, Mercieca sent three-person teams of Army and Navy personnel out to the most distressed hospitals to go through that hospital's roster of patients and select those who met the Javits admission criteria.

Dr. Deborah Salas-Lopez, who worked at Javits with Mercieca and her team, observed that initially there was a communications issue. "The fact that many hospitals were operating in crisis mode didn't help the situation as they had little time to understand what was being built at Javits and how it could help them [transfer] patients," she wrote in a report. "Initially, some hospitals refused to let the liaison officers come to them, claiming they had no time or space to give them. After explaining what we could do to help them, they relented and allowed for the liaisons to come to them."

When Mercieca and colleagues started work at the Javits Center, there were ten patients total and 990 empty beds. And it had taken ten days to reach even that number. By changing from a push to a pull approach, Javits went from taking ten patients total in ten days to admitting 120 patients a day during the peak. The

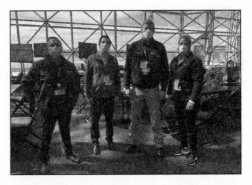

Pictured are just a few of the Northwell operations team members at Javits.

census went from ten to 465 in three weeks. Included within the Javits were forty-eight ICU beds in case patients deteriorated during their stay there. Most patients got much better, but there were some whose condition spiraled just when it seemed they were recovering. "That's part of this disease," said Mercieca. "They're okay and then they become short of breath, their saturation drops, and if you're not with them they die."

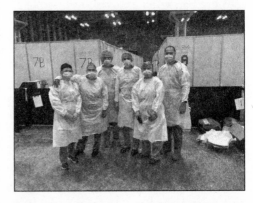

Pictured are clinical staff members who treated patients at Javits.

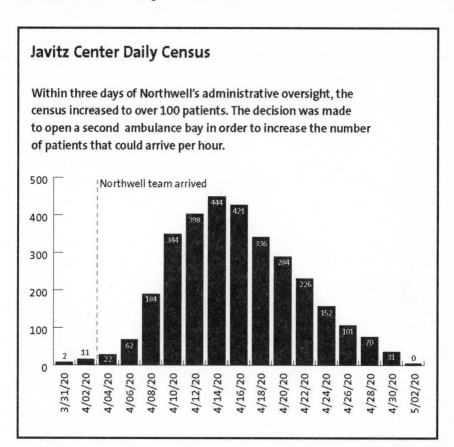

Javitz Center Daily Census

Within three days of Northwell's administrative oversight, the census increased to over 100 patients. The decision was made to open a second ambulance bay in order to increase the number of patients that could arrive per hour.

With more patients coming in, the Javits Center required more doctors to facilitate the admitting process. A number of hospitals sent physicians in to help, and we had one physician from Northwell, Dr. Eric Cruzen, admit patients from all twenty-three of our hospitals—approving those who needed to be moved, bypassing red tape, and moving patients rapidly to an open Javits bed. Mercieca urged the other major New York health systems to send a representative to work in a similar fashion on behalf of their hospitals. Representatives came from New York Presbyterian, Mt. Sinai, and the New York City public hospital system. At the same time, the three-person Army and Navy teams visited more stand-alone and distressed hospitals to identify patients eligible for transfer to Javits.

Rita Mercieca and her team worked fourteen- and fifteen-hour days for twenty-six of the twenty-eight days they were at Javits until the last patient was discharged on Mercieca's twenty-eighth day there. During that time, the vast majority of patients recovered. Patients were tested on a regular basis to determine their oxygen level, and a patient who could maintain a healthy oxygen level while walking across the Javits Center—about six hundred feet up and back—was eligible for discharge. That key part of the discharge process was referred to by the military as the "walk of life." "The walk of life happened like this," explained Mercieca. "They would take the oxygen off the patient and somebody would accompany them and walk them across the Javits, which is like walking across a football field, and see how they did. If they became short of breath or if their oxygen dropped below a certain number, they would fail the walk of life. If they passed the walk of life, they would go home."

In retrospect, Mercieca believes a lot of excellent work was done at Javits. She also believes that the *Comfort* took a lot of heat for starting out with a prohibition against taking COVID patients, but she notes that the *Comfort* wound up taking extremely sick patients into their ICU and sending the rest to Javits. "One night, Jamaica Hospital had a problem with their oxygen supplies and the *Comfort* took ten of their ICU patients. I'm talking about really sick ICU patients, ten of them, in two hours." Maybe saving ten lives in that one night. In all, the *Comfort* proved helpful by seeing a total of 182 patients.

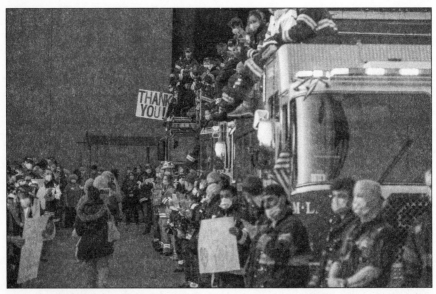

Just one example of the gratitude expressed at the 7 p.m. shift change at one of our Northwell hospitals.

CHAPTER SEVEN

Policy and Regulation—
The Government's Role

Lessons
- Many government rules and regulations concerning health care are unnecessary.
- The innovation resulting from the relaxation of many government rules is an indication that many of those rules should be reviewed and possibly changed in the future.
- Government leadership is essential to provide both policy guidance and response coordination while refraining from micromanagement.
- Strong professional relationships with elected officials and regulators enable faster action during a crisis.
- There is an urgent need to strengthen the ability of safety net hospitals and ambulatory providers to cope with major disasters.

With Governor Cuomo as the quarterback of the New York State response to the pandemic, state government played a pivotal role in our ability to adapt to the crisis. Among the central lessons we take from the experience is that when government regulators waive multiple laws and regulations, we are free to adapt to the crisis more readily. In many respects, the governor was a partner with Northwell and all other health care providers in this endeavor. He provided clarity and sensible direction throughout, took tough stands when needed, and made decisions based on science and data. Strong professional relationships make a difference in a crisis, as we noted in chapter 5 when we reported on the significance of relationships with vendors of PPE and other equipment. A similar principle applies to relationships with government officials. There are times when the relationships between health systems and government regulators are contentious. Regulators want to know we are playing by the rules. At the same time, we need the freedom in our hospitals and ambulatory sites to take care of patients in a way that is consistent with our own best judgment. The goal is to find a reasonable balance where laws and regulations protect consumers from bad actors while, at the same time, the vast majority of honorable clinicians are given appropriate freedom to practice in a way that best serves patients. We learned during the crisis that many regulations are overly prescriptive and many just plain out of date with the progression of medical science. The commissioner of the state Department of Health, Dr. Howard Zucker, understood this and was essential throughout the crisis in helping all provider organizations have the ability to operate without undue constraints.

As we have noted, the key to all of the regulatory relief was a decision by Governor Cuomo to declare a state of emergency in New York, an action that triggered a series of emergency powers permitting him to suspend existing laws. The Albany *Times Union* reported that the governor changed 262 laws over a fifty-five-day period. In February, before the first case of COVID was discovered in New York State, the governor asked the legislature to grant him broad authority to make whatever changes were necessary in the emergency to protect the health and lives of New Yorkers.

A word about relationships: It so happened in this case that one of us (Michael Dowling) had known Governor Cuomo for several decades. He had, in fact, worked for Andrew Cuomo's father Mario Cuomo when the latter was governor of New York during the 1980s and 1990s. Dowling served as one of Mario Cuomo's closest advisors in government and remained a close friend for the rest of Mario Cuomo's life. Knowing Andrew Cuomo as Michael Dowling does made communication between the two men easy and comfortable. Long-standing mutual trust between the two men anchored the relationship in the crisis.

* * *

Alexandra Trinkoff, vice president of legal affairs at Northwell, saw early on that there were multiple roadblocks in state and federal regulations and laws that had the potential of preventing us from providing care to an unpredictable influx of patients. For example, our surge plans called for treating patients in areas in our hospitals where regulations prohibited doing so. Our staffing plans called for hiring out-of-state nurses, physicians, and other providers to pitch in, which is prohibited and subject to criminal and civil liability without a specific New York State license. But new problems require new rules.

At the start of the emergency, but before the peak, Trinkoff started to build a database of the various issues where she expected we would need relief from state or federal rules. We worked together with the state, the Greater New York Hospital Association, and the Hospital Association of New York to inform officials that relief from existing rules would better enable us to fight the virus. Trinkoff and her team created a searchable PDF which included every executive order from state and federal government and all orders and advisory opinions from any regulatory agency that might affect what we could or could not do at Northwell. This was a modest document in the early days, but an indication of the size and complexity of the crisis is that it grew to 250 single-spaced pages in a matter of weeks. Trinkoff worked with Dennis Whalen, Northwell vice president of government affairs, and connected with key people throughout our health system to put together requests for waivers to state and federal agencies. Officials at both levels were accommodating from the start. A key waiver came early when the state ruled that doctors from other states were exempt from the rule requiring a New York license. Trinkoff and other Northwell team members went back to the state and asked for a similar ruling for nurses and respiratory therapists and it was granted, which enabled our system to hire additional staff from many different states. The state would give a little at a time in terms of waivers and exemptions and then, by mid-March when the virus struck, scores of waivers each day would come in from local, state, and federal government, as well as from regulatory agencies such as the New York State Department of Health, the Centers for Medicare and Medicaid Services, the CDC, and FDA. The waivers and guidance covered everything from providing legal immunity to clinical staff in the hospitals to allowing recent graduates of medical and nursing schools to immediately practice in the hospital without going through the normal licensing process. In many cases, regulatory restrictions that we and other health systems have strained against for years were suspended. including elaborate certificate-of-need applications any time a health system wishes to expand its footprint or services. It freed our organization to care for very sick patients.

Perhaps the most important ruling came from the state government to indemnify physicians and other clinicians working in the crisis. The legislature followed up by giving this indemnification the force of law. As we noted in chapter 6, the move enabled physicians unaccustomed to working at the front lines of a public health emergency to do so. Hundreds of our doctors were eager to volunteer but they quite reasonably conveyed the caveat that they would be unable to do so unless they were protected from being sued by a patient and from criminal liability for performing tasks in a setting such as an ICU which was outside of everyday practice. Relaxed rules concerning scope of practice allowed clinicians to work at the top of their licenses by eliminating certain supervision requirements for certain types of providers, like nurse practitioners and physician assistants, and also provided the necessary staff to care for the influx of patients, which at times exceeded 100 percent of the hospitals' licensed capacity.

Many of the laws and regulations are excessive to begin with. For example, there is a provision in New York that prevents a licensed clinician from working in alternative locations—such as in a tent on the North Shore University Hospital campus or in the Javits Center. Jeff Kraut, Northwell executive vice president for strategy and analytics, noted that there were good reasons for the existence of many rules, but they are outdated today. For example, New York historically had higher standards than some other states for physician practices and thus did not grant licensed out-of-state doctors the ability to practice in New York without going through the New York licensing process. In times past, it was often impossible to determine whether a particular physician had a history of disciplinary actions for malpractice or inappropriate behavior. But with a national database, that is no longer a concern.

One of the most important rule changes—and we hope among the most sustainable—concerned telehealth. The New York State Department of Financial Services followed the lead of the Centers for Medicare and Medicaid Services, the federal agency that administers Medicare, in saying that insurance plans should pay for telehealth visits at the same rate as they pay for in-person visits. This is essential to the success of telehealth. If telehealth interactions between patients and doctors are paid at a lower rate, doctors would lose substantial revenue on those transactions, disrupting the financial viability of primary care practices in particular. More than that, the government loosened restrictions on the type of software that could be used in telehealth visits. Said Trinkoff: "The federal government decided 'we don't care whether it's HIPAA compliant. If you can do a telehealth visit on Skype or on FaceTime, that is acceptable during the period that the national emergency is in effect." Telehealth raises sensitive issues around HIPAA regulations, which were written at a time prior to the widespread use of texting. Under HIPAA rules, we at Northwell are not permitted to send a text message to a patient reminding them to fill out a particular form. This sort of regulation serves no purpose other than to prevent people from using the simple technology they rely on for so much else in their lives.

Other key exemptions to existing laws and rules involved the use of space. Governments tend to micromanage how different kinds of spaces in hospitals and nursing homes can be used. The governor asked every hospital in the state to try and double patient capacity. Under normal rules, this would involve navigating a regulatory maze and take years to accomplish. But with a stroke of his pen Governor Cuomo allowed us to implement our surge plans, which enabled us to do exactly what he asked us to do—dramatically increase bed capacity. "We looked at things completely differently," said Trinkoff. "It was almost as if you were given a new set of eyes. You saw conference rooms that were too small to meet regulatory requirements, where you would never be permitted to put patients. All of a sudden that didn't matter anymore. As long as you had enough oxygen and electricity to support the ventilators, you could use that space."

Most of these rules are designed for patient safety. You don't want people cutting corners or having unsafe fire safety plans in a place where you are putting hospital patients. You want to make sure that there's enough oxygen and airflow, backup power and other requirements. "But what we learned," said Trinkoff, "is that hospitals are pretty good at creating space that's going to work for the disease, and that maybe if you set the parameters, the hospitals can self-police and we can move and adapt in a more efficient manner to meet patient care needs," rather than having to file massive amounts of paperwork to satisfy regulators.

* * *

The good news is that the government recognized that during this crisis those of us in the medical community needed flexibility to do our jobs, and that when we got that flexibility we were able to do many different things that saved lives. Which raises an important question as to what to do after the crisis is over: What are the essential lessons learned relating to what extent government should regulate doctors and hospitals? Whatever the precise nature of statutory or regulatory revisions, Jeff Kraut believes there should be an emergency act at the ready which grants the governor the broad powers he had during the pandemic. To streamline the process, said Kraut, there should be a single executive order that allows scores or even hundreds of suspensions of rules and laws to kick in.

In a broader sense, reverting to the pre-pandemic regulatory status quo would be a mistake. Along with other hospitals and physician groups, we are in the process of working with regulators to identify rules—especially those long on the books—that do little more than thwart the ability of doctors and hospitals to do their work. Bureaucracies can be stubborn forces blocking change. Said Trinkoff: "What we've seen after almost every major public health emergency has been increased regulatory scrutiny." After Hurricane Sandy, for example, "people forgot that we saved lives; essentially evacuated a five-hundred-person hospital in eight hours before it lost power. They don't really remember that. But they remember that you were provided thirty million dollars in FEMA funding and you didn't save your receipts."

Medicare rules, for example, are so complex and confusing that Trinkoff and her colleagues needed a detailed chart to determine whether a telehealth visit between a doctor and patient could be billed to Medicare. When most of the rules were thrown out the window during the crisis, doctors and hospitals responded well. The case for restoring all the previous rules seems tenuous.

"We're hoping the pendulum will swing back from the state micro-managing low-value activities that are not directly related to quality patient care," said Jeff Kraut. The amount of documentation doctors and nurses are required to do, for example, reduces the time they can spend taking care of patients, and while a certain degree of documentation on patient treatment is helpful, the burden has grown over the years to a counterproductive level. During the crisis, said Kraut, we "were relieved of many low value administrative requirements. We'd like to see some of those things revisited to reduce the administrative burden." We think it would also be beneficial for the state to work with providers to determine the data that should be reported to the state and its form—a uniform standard across the board would reduce bureaucracy.

Dennis Whalen has had a front-row seat in Albany observing changes in laws and regulations related to health care, and he has seen a definite shift over time that constricts the ability of health-care professionals to do their jobs. This is not to suggest that there is not an important over-sight role for government in the health-care space. But if this crisis proves anything, it is that greater flexibility allows doctors, nurses, and other clinicians to provide care in a faster, more effective manner when regu-latory constraints are loosened. An example involves constraints on how beds can be used or where in a hospital patients may be treated. With COVID-19 those rules were thrown out the window and for very good reason. We needed to treat patients in lobbies, conference rooms, audi-toriums: anywhere we could place a bed. These were lifesaving actions. In an emergency, we need the flexibility to be able to care for patients in whatever area of our hospitals we can find for them. Under state rules, for example, pediatric beds cannot be used for adults, but in a particu-larly tough flu season we have more sick people than we can handle in our adult beds but few children. Shouldn't we have the flexibility under emergency circumstances to place adults in pediatric units? "It's not uncommon during the flu season for us to have thirty, forty, fifty people waiting for a bed because we can only put them in this type of bed," said Kraut. "Well, what we learned with COVID is that we can adequately care for people if you give us the freedom to decide how to use our facility when those spikes occur."

* * *

A major issue raised during the pandemic concerned equity. In late April 2020, a *New York Times* article reported that "The coronavirus recession has exacerbated the racial and income divides in America."* Earlier that month the head of the California Health Care Foundation wrote that "the pandemic has created a perfect storm of irrefutable evidence that people of color are caught in a web of social inequality." We knew from firsthand experience that large numbers of our patients at Forest Hills Hospital, for example, were from low-income families in crowded urban neighborhoods. As we reflect upon the experience of dealing with the COVID outbreak in New York, there are difficult questions that those of us in the health-care community as well as in government must face up to. Were there inequities in access to care among rich and poor? Were there inequities in access to high quality care? What must we as a society do in the months and years ahead to provide the best possible care to people living in communities that took a disproportionate brunt of the damage from the coronavirus? The dedicated clinicians at New York's public hospitals do heroic work for their patients, but too often these facilities are underfunded. The challenges at Elmhurst Hospital that we noted in chapter 2 were widely covered in the news media. Elmhurst is part of the New York City public hospital system, but the situation there amid the crisis calls into question the use of the word *system*. For it seemed, at least part of the time, that the clinicians at Elmhurst lacked a safety valve to load balance patients into other facilities. And we know

---

* Jim Tankersley, "Job or Health? Restarting the Economy Threatens to Worsen Economic Inequality," *New York Times*, April 27, 2020.

from our own experience that there was significant pressure put on the staff and facilities at Jamaica Hospital, a neighboring safety net provider. If the public system in New York City requires a greater investment to improve infrastructure and capacity, then we have an obligation as a society to make that investment.

At Northwell we take our responsibility to care for patients in underserved areas very seriously. We have been asked by the state to help do exactly that in many ways at many times. In 2019, our team at Northwell dug into a complex set of problems and produced a detailed study of how to save four community hospitals in central Brooklyn that were facing dire financial realities (Brookdale, Wykoff, Kingsbrook, and Interfaith). At the governor's request, one of us (Michael Dowling) has cochaired the last two commissions established to help solve the state's Medicaid budget problem. There are ways in which we consider ourselves an extension of the state government, and comfortably so. A number of our top executives worked for the state in various capacities. Some did so under the administration of Governor Mario Cuomo while others worked under more recent governors. Our Northwell state government veterans include Michael Dowling, Mark Solazzo, Head of Contracting Howard Gold, Communications Chief Terry Lynam, Chief Strategist Jeff Kraut, and Government Relations Head Dennis Whalen.

Questions about disparities in health care in our country are certainly not new. But it is more urgent now than ever to address the problem in light of the combined tragedies of the pandemic as well as the killings of Black people by police. How can we better serve all people, including those in underserved communities? Certainly one step is to prepare for the next viral assault. More than that, though, is the need to rethink the way we deliver care in minority areas so that we provide better access when people are sick, but that we also work more proactively than ever to go back upstream and provide the kind of preventive services that head off illness in the first place. This is where a great opportunity lies.

All of us in the health-care realm—whether in provider organizations or government—have a responsibility in the time ahead to think about how to make sure that facilities that disproportionately serve low-income neighborhoods and people of color are every bit as high quality and adaptable as Forest Hills proved to be at the height of the crisis.

How do you make sure poorer communities are as well taken care of as affluent communities? Dennis Whalen noted that at Northwell we are a "self-contained system; we can independently make these decisions and decide where we're going to move resources from here to there." In government, however, he notes that there are layers of hierarchy and bureaucracy that often prevent seamless decision-making and action. And, crucially, governments are not free to spend money on what they chose to improve at any given time. Public hospitals, said Whalen, "are hamstrung, because it's not a true system."

In New York, there is a good foundational relationship between the governor and leaders of major health systems. In the months ahead there will be discussions about how to create a state of overall readiness for next time that makes sure no one is left behind. These issues and many others are being explored by a number of leaders who have been asked by the governor to help to reimagine the future of New York post-COVID. Among those involved in this initiative is Eric Schmidt, former CEO of Google, along with Mike Bloomberg and the Gates Foundation. In addition, one of us (Michael Dowling) was asked by the governor to help reimagine the future of health-care delivery in the state. In practice, this effort will involve defining the lessons learned from the crisis and preparing for the next time, so that when future leaders face a similar crisis, they will have the benefit of general guidance as well as blueprints for how to prepare.

Whatever the plan for a future pandemic, a major lesson this time was that while state officials have knowledge about policy and regulation, their actions must be coordinated with people on the front lines who are actually doing the work. Those of us in the business of treating patients every day have the experience and knowledge both to understand what must be done, and to make it happen.

CHAPTER EIGHT

Research Trials—
The Rigor of Science

Lessons
- Having a major research institute within a system enables you to conduct clinical trials quickly and with scientific rigor.
- A global pandemic is a call to action for scientists to generate reliable data and convey a message of hope to patients and doctors.
- The volume of information resulting from our having treated so many COVID patients created an enormous database for future research and study.
- Political leaders would advance the cause of science by sticking to the data rather than speculating about the efficacy of largely untested methods.
- Science in the United States is underfunded and under-respected. The danger posed by political leaders with little understanding of science cannot be overstated.

"We're facing a disease for which there's no treatment," said Dr. Kevin Tracey, a neurosurgeon who heads the Feinstein Institutes for Medical Research at Northwell. "Think of what that means. We're ramping up with preparations to have the hospitals filled up with people in every bed.

Some of them dying of a disease, surrounded by doctors and nurses who don't know what to do because they have never seen the disease. No one has the treatment."

The situation, said Tracey, is a tragedy. For a medical researcher, it also creates an obligation because "this is a research problem." And a piece of a potential solution lay all around Tracey in Northwell's twenty-three hospitals, which were about to be full of very sick COVID patients—a unique frontline setting for scientific testing. At Northwell, we were in the US epicenter, and others who would later experience the virus would be learning from what we did. Our obligation was to research and educate.

On Friday, March 13, as the virus swept into the New York area, Tracey made the decision to set up a series of COVID clinical trials to better understand the virus and search for therapies. Tracey and his Feinstein Institutes colleagues Meredith Burcyk and Jon Cohen, along

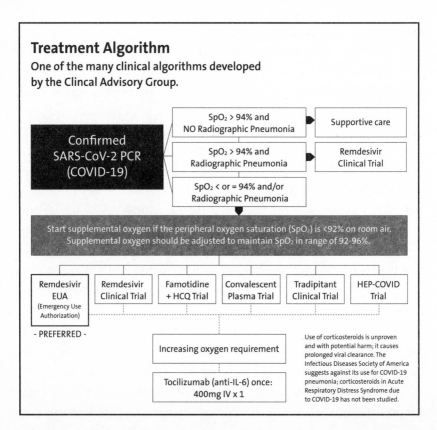

Treatment Algorithm
One of the many clinical algorithms developed by the Clincal Advisory Group.

Confirmed SARS-CoV-2 PCR (COVID-19)

- SpO_2 > 94% and NO Radiographic Pneumonia → Supportive care
- SpO_2 > 94% and Radiographic Pneumonia → Remdesivir Clinical Trial
- SpO_2 < or = 94% and/or Radiographic Pneumonia

Start supplemental oxygen if the peripheral oxygen saturation (SpO_2) is <92% on room air. Supplemental oxygen should be adjusted to maintain SpO_2 in range of 92-96%.

| Remdesivir EUA (Emergency Use Authorization) | Remdesivir Clinical Trial | Famotidine + HCQ Trial | Convalescent Plasma Trial | Tradipitant Clinical Trial | HEP-COVID Trial |

- PREFERRED -

Increasing oxygen requirement

Tocilizumab (anti-IL-6) once: 400mg IV x 1

Use of corticosteroids is unproven and with potential harm; it causes prolonged viral clearance. The Infectious Diseases Society of America suggests against its use for COVID-19 pneumonia; corticosteroids in Acute Respiratory Distress Syndrome due to COVID-19 has not been studied.

with Dr. Christina Brennan as the medical leader, established the outlines of a COVID clinical trials unit within Feinstein with two objec-
tives: "To produce reliable data through rigorous scientific research and
to send a message of hope to patients and doctors that we are working
on it." By May 1, we had started six different trials and enrolled over 850
patients with support from more than two hundred investigators, coordinators, nurses, and other personnel.

Redeployment of the troops, which had been so important in the
medical units, would work in research as well. Many Feinstein researchers had been running clinical trials on other medical questions, but their
patients were unavailable—since the hospitals had been cleared of just
about everyone except COVID patients—putting those trials on hold.
That freed up a number of scientists who Tracey recruited to start looking into aspects of the coronavirus.

By the end of the day that Friday, the plans were laid out, and by
the next morning, the team went about executing it. We were fortunate
to have Tracey in this role leading the research. He had long ago established himself as one of the elite biomedical researchers in the world,
with expertise in the areas of inflammation, sepsis, and the neuroscience
of immunity. He had made a particularly important contribution in creating an essentially new field known as bioelectronic medicine, and, with
his colleagues, developing devices to replace anti-inflammatory drugs in
clinical trials of rheumatoid arthritis. Clinical trials of this work have
enabled some patients with crippling inflammatory diseases to regain a
significant degree of movement and overall health.

In setting up coronavirus trials, Tracey worked with Drs. Mark
Jarrett, David Battinelli, and Thomas McGinn on the logistics for
such research. As Mark Jarrett said, it was important to move quickly.
One of the most important lessons of the crisis, said Jarrett, is to "get
patients into studies as quickly as possible. By spring we had so many
sick patients that we were an ideal location for trials, and we engaged in
a number of these, testing different potential remedies. It was important
to try and get eligible patients into the trials because we were hungry for
data on what might actually work."

There are some potential treatments for COVID-19 that, while
unproven, possess certain antiviral properties that make them worth

trying. Some of these potential remedies are drugs that were developed to treat other conditions, but that scientists think may possibly work on the coronavirus. There was an air of desperation among patients, doctors, and researchers that pervaded the search for a treatment, given the nature of the situation. It is very difficult for doctors to tell patients who are close to dying that there is nothing to be done. "We all understand the 'compassionate use' issues of medications and treatments," said Jarrett, "but, a vast majority of our patients should be in studies looking at these drugs because in this case we may get a second peak in the late fall, early winter that could be worse than this peak."

The idea was to conduct gold-standard trials and share knowledge with the world. "We committed to a path of scientific rigor, ethical and regulatory compliance, FDA oversight, and sponsorship," said Tracey. "We focused on randomized clinical trials. If we learned something, the rest of the world would also learn from what we learned. We committed to this path from day zero. We didn't want to get into this chaos of anecdotes that was created around hydroxychloroquine and other things."

Having been involved in scores of trials through the years and authoring more than 350 research papers, Tracey was well-known throughout the pharmaceutical world. On Saturday morning, March 14, he reached out to scientists he knew at the biopharmaceutical companies on the forefront of COVID research, Regeneron and Gilead. Regeneron had been studying interleukin 6 inhibitors (IL-6) and Gilead was starting trials on a new antiviral drug called Remdesivir. He connected with the chief medical officer at Regeneron on Saturday and they agreed that Northwell would conduct a trial to test whether their product, sarilumab, an IL-6 inhibitor, would be effective in preventing damaging inflammation during COVID. Tracey told the Regeneron official that he would work with them on a trial if Regeneron would "commit to telling me that you have drug available, and that your team will work nonstop until we get the patients treated in the next few days. Because we have people dying in our hospitals and they have no drugs." Teams from Regeneron, Northwell, and the FDA worked through that March weekend and by Monday Tracey and colleagues were reviewing a research protocol. The process of setting up a trial and treating the first patient normally takes two or three months. In this instance the Northwell and Regeneron teams had done it in three days.

We moved quickly recruiting patients. In a typical clinical trial about five to ten patients per year are enrolled. On the Regeneron trial at Northwell we enrolled 216 patients in a few weeks thanks to the work of the COVID clinical trials unit and the principal investigator, Negin Hajizadeh. "It takes hours of work to screen people, get them enrolled, give the drug in the right way, at the right time," said Tracey. "We had a small army of people now working on about six clinical trials at five of our major hospitals: Staten Island, Lenox Hill, North Shore, Long Island Jewish, and Northern Westchester." Of the first four hundred patients in the Regeneron trial, 226 were at Northwell hospitals.

To be eligible for the trial, patients had to have severe pneumonia and low blood oxygen. They also had to be hospitalized and progressing toward needing a ventilator but not yet intubated, or in the ICU and already on a ventilator. "These were extremely sick people," said Tracey. Deciding whether to participate in a trial made for highly emotional decisions by patients' families. Doctors explained to them that number one, the trial drug might not work, and number two, their loved one might get a placebo instead of the drug being tested.

The trial was barely a few weeks old when, suddenly in early April, Regeneron froze the initiative. The company was reviewing data from the first wave of the trial and aiming to reopen it with a larger group. But the data, said Tracey, was disappointing. The remedy was not working in early-stage patients, causing Regeneron to switch gears and focus the trial on only the very sickest patients.

Tracey, along with colleagues Drs. Marcia Epstein and Prasat Malhotra, also worked with Gilead Sciences on a trial for the drug Remdesivir. Tracey agreed to enter into the trials knowing it involved a significant amount of work for the already overworked Northwell staff, but he is a scientist first and foremost and sought a path to study possible therapies in a rigorous way. He was emphatic with Gilead, as he had been with Regeneron, that they would do the trials on one condition: "Our patients are dying, and I need you to tell me you are going to send me as much drug as I can use." Regeneron had followed through on this commitment, but Gilead never sent more than a few doses at a time, frustrating Tracey and his team. At Northwell we enrolled only a fraction of the patients we could have included in the Gilead trial due to the limited supply of the drug made available to us.

* * *

One of the most significant research efforts globally of the coronavirus is the initiative at Northwell led by Dr. Thomas McGinn, Northwell deputy physician-in-chief, and Karina Davidson, senior vice president of research at Northwell. They built a data consortium of 140 data experts and clinical specialists. This capability was constructed in a two-week period during the COVID crisis in New York and has resulted in what McGinn describes as "the world's largest COVID database." A by-product of New York having been the epicenter of the pandemic in the United States is that McGinn, Davidson, and their team have virtually every conceivable data point on 16,655 in-patients. The team published the first significant study of COVID in the *Journal of the American Medical Association* (*JAMA*) at the height of the crisis in New York. That study, by lead author Dr. Safiya Richardson and a number of colleagues,

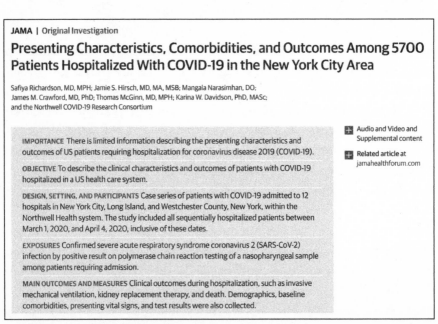

JAMA | Original Investigation

Presenting Characteristics, Comorbidities, and Outcomes Among 5700 Patients Hospitalized With COVID-19 in the New York City Area

Safiya Richardson, MD, MPH; Jamie S. Hirsch, MD, MA, MSB; Mangala Narasimhan, DO; James M. Crawford, MD, PhD; Thomas McGinn, MD, MPH; Karina W. Davidson, PhD, MASc; and the Northwell COVID-19 Research Consortium

➕ Audio and Video and Supplemental content

➕ Related article at jamahealthforum.com

IMPORTANCE There is limited information describing the presenting characteristics and outcomes of US patients requiring hospitalization for coronavirus disease 2019 (COVID-19).

OBJECTIVE To describe the clinical characteristics and outcomes of patients with COVID-19 hospitalized in a US health care system.

DESIGN, SETTING, AND PARTICIPANTS Case series of patients with COVID-19 admitted to 12 hospitals in New York City, Long Island, and Westchester County, New York, within the Northwell Health system. The study included all sequentially hospitalized patients between March 1, 2020, and April 4, 2020, inclusive of these dates.

EXPOSURES Confirmed severe acute respiratory syndrome coronavirus 2 (SARS-CoV-2) infection by positive result on polymerase chain reaction testing of a nasopharyngeal sample among patients requiring admission.

MAIN OUTCOMES AND MEASURES Clinical outcomes during hospitalization, such as invasive mechanical ventilation, kidney replacement therapy, and death. Demographics, baseline comorbidities, presenting vital signs, and test results were also collected.

This research conducted by Northwell became the lead article in *JAMA*.

including McGinn and Davidson, found that significant comorbidities were present in large numbers of COVID-19 patients. The study found, for example, that the most common comorbidities in the 5,700 patients studied were "hypertension (57 percent), obesity (41 percent), and diabetes (34 percent). . . . Patients with diabetes were more likely to have received invasive mechanical ventilation, received treatment in the intensive care unit or developed acute kidney disease."

These important findings revealed that a combination of lifestyle and preexisting conditions are factors in determining who succumbs to the virus. "The vast majority of deaths from this virus are of the elderly, the obese, the diabetic, and the hypertensives," said Tracey. "And many of the hypertensives are the obese diabetics. So, yes, we've all seen the terrible stories on the news of the young healthy athlete who dropped dead suddenly of COVID, but demographics and genetics influence outcomes. You have a disproportionate number of underserved people who have a higher incidence of hypertension and obesity as well."

McGinn noted that this was "the largest description of any group of COVID patients in the world." In 2020 alone the research consortium had more than twenty research papers either published or in preparation for publication. Among those papers was a study examining the evidence on whether patients were more likely to survive with early intubation or delaying intubation. This critical work will help clinicians gain a better understanding of when and under what conditions patients should be placed on ventilators. Another examines the deleterious impact of COVID on kidney function and yet another explores the dangerous effects of COVID on blood clotting. Patients in these studies will be followed through 2022 for an extensive longitudinal study in a major effort to learn the longer-term effects of COVID.

* * *

During the week of March 17, while working on both the Regeneron and Gilead trials, Tracey received a call from a physician colleague he had known for twenty-plus years. Dr. Michael Callahan, who had been at the meeting Dr. Tracey attended twenty years earlier advising defense department officials about preparing for a pandemic, and who was in China during the coronavirus outbreak, told Tracey that there was some important data that might hold a clue for a new trial. It seemed that patients in China who had been diagnosed with acid reflux (heartburn) fared far better when infected by the virus than others. What was different about these patients was that all were taking famotidine for their reflux disease, an over-the-counter drug sold under a variety of brand names, including Pepcid.

Dr. Callahan said he understood that we at Northwell were getting "slammed" by the pandemic and Dr. Tracey explained that we had many people dying in our hospitals and no proven therapies with which to treat them. Callahan explained what the data in China showed about patients on famotidine. He added that computer modeling indicated it was possible famotidine interacts with one of the virus proteins and while they didn't know if that would kill the virus, a study was reasonable. The COVID clinical trials unit went to work setting up the trial.

At HHS, Robert Kadlec, assistant secretary for preparedness and response at the US Department of Health & Human Services, asked Tracey to move quickly to conduct a research study into the efficacy of famotidine as a therapy for COVID-19. The trial, led by principal investigator Dr. Joseph Conigliaro, commenced on April 7 after Northwell quietly purchased a significant supply of the drug. This took time in light of the fact that the trial required an injectable form of famotidine, which is rarely used, so that hospitalized patients could be given the drug intravenously. The study was funded by a contract from the Biomedical Advanced Research and Development Authority (BARDA).

Tracey was pleased to have the study up and running, but it was not exactly an ideal study in his view. Politics had interfered with the shape of the trial. President Trump's insistent promotion of hydroxychloroquine as a remedy had influenced patients and doctors to demand the drug. This was an unfortunate situation. There was no scientific evidence that hydroxychloroquine could work but the president had been promoting it nonetheless. Worse still, a later study on hydroxychloroquine in April was halted when it was learned that some patients had developed irregular heart rhythms while on the drug. Nonetheless, at the time the famotidine trial began, hydroxychloroquine had suddenly become the current "standard of care" and therefore had to be tested along with famotidine.

In an April 26 article in *Science* magazine, Tracey was quoted on the matter: "Is it good science? No. It's the real world." And in the real world there would be no pure trial comparing famotidine to a placebo. Instead, the trial would test famotidine plus hydroxychloroquine or hydroxychloroquine alone. "The reason for hydroxychloroquine as spelled out in the documents," said Tracey, "is that hydroxychloroquine was the standard of care because the president said it would work, so patients and families followed suit." Tracey's Northwell colleague Dr. McGinn said there was no scientific evidence to suggest hydroxychloroquine might work other than a small French study that was poorly done in that it evaluated forty patients in a non-randomized way. Even that study showed minimal benefit if any. "Anybody that knows anything about randomized trials, control trials, knows it was just crap," said McGinn. "And that became counted as the only drug that works. It should have gone to a larger, randomized trial to prove benefit. But, you know, on the other hand, people were desperate. They wanted something. Their loved ones were dying." Tracey judged the French study "a complete failure."

As Tracey put it, "the standard of care was determined by politics." Then suddenly, in the midst of the trial of hydroxychloroquine with and without famotidine, hydroxychloroquine was judged to no longer be the "standard of care." The new standard would be Remdesivir, based on comments by Dr. Anthony Fauci that it had demonstrated some clinical value.

As of July 10 when the book went to press the results of the famotidine trial were being analyzed.

* * *

Tracey worries that science in the United States is "under siege. It has been underfunded and underappreciated for decades." And at the height of the pandemic a drug becomes the "standard of care" because the president speculates, without any scientific evidence, that it might work. Has respect for science eroded over the years? Tracey believes it has, and he holds out hope that the coronavirus pandemic may be a wakeup call or, as he put it, a "Sputnik event," referring to when American scientists accelerated the space race after the Russians launched Sputnik.

"If you want a cure for COVID-19, fund science," he said. "Not with a stimulus package. Make up for the seventeen years of scientific funding in the US not keeping up with inflation. There has got to be a reality check that this will happen again unless we make the right investments in our scientific infrastructure. Scientific infrastructure can eliminate this disease."

Scientific history is instructive here, he said:

Look at the history of the human race. What have we done with viruses? We've thrown major resources at the problem. Polio: decades of investment by the March of Dimes, decades of investment by the government funded laboratories. Look at HIV: billions of dollars thrown at the problem, but thrown at the problem with scientific rigor and people, including Dr. Fauci, who were supported and celebrated.

This response has to be like the response to Sputnik. So a few months before I was born, Sputnik was sailing over Earth, and people were listening to it on their radios—beep, beep, beep—and it scared the shit out of the United States. And soon after JFK stood up and said, we're going to go to the moon and back. And what you saw was a sustained effort and an investment in science that created me and everybody else in my generation. This vision of scientific excellence has been pummeled in the last twenty years. We need to have a sustained investment in research that gets us back to the levels of before seventeen years ago. And then we have to keep ahead of inflation if we want to stay ahead in our science. Right now, whether it's China, Israel, Germany, Sweden, or the UK, these countries are eating our lunch in terms of investment in research for their universities and institutes as a percentage of GDP. They're eating our lunch.

CHAPTER NINE

Communications—Information Is Healthy, Fear Is Not

Lessons
- In a crisis, information is healthy, fear is not.
- A public health crisis creates an opportunity to engage with consumers and the public about taking action steps to improve their health.
- Be prepared to engage with the media—print, online, radio, and TV—and be as transparent as possible in sharing information. While it must be controlled and managed, strong news media engagement helps educate the public during a public health emergency.
- Continuous internal communications provide employees with facts needed to understand the reality of the situation. It cannot be overdone.
- Leadership must provide a sense of calm, confidence, and optimism. Project a winning attitude.
- Leadership must be visible—face-to-face encounters are important.

In the early stages of the pandemic, we had many more questions than answers. As the coronavirus was making its way from Asia to Europe and the United States, we did not know much about it. The Chinese had been opaque at best. There were no rigorous studies out of China that could guide us. Early on we did not know that many infected people were asymptomatic. We did not know about the kidney damage and blood clotting that accompanied many cases. We did not know that loss of a sense of taste and smell could be early clues, or how the virus would manifest in children through a condition known as multisystem inflammatory syndrome. We certainly did not know about the destructive speed with which the virus assaulted its victims. We did not know that patients with preexisting conditions such as heart disease, diabetes, and obesity would prove to be far more vulnerable to COVID-19.

What we did know from day one, however, was that at Northwell we had a responsibility to serve as a trusted source of information and guidance to the communities we serve in the New York region; and that we would use the medical and scientific resources within Northwell to inform the public at every step. The perfect storm of widespread ignorance about the virus plus a tremendous hunger among the public for information made this a communications challenge unlike anything we had ever experienced. But communication is an essential element within our emergency response capability and we acted quickly.

Chief Marketing and Communications Officer Ramon Soto and his team huddled with clinical and administrative leaders early on to try and understand what lay ahead and how Northwell's communications capabilities could be helpful to the public as well as our own employees. "We spent a lot of time with the docs to understand this new thing. How is it going to progress through society?" said Soto. "What does the curve look like? And what are the challenges at each stage of the curve?" As Soto and colleagues Terry Lynam, Barbara Osborn, and Tom Sclafani were learning and preparing, it became clear that New York was the epicenter within the United States and Northwell the epicenter within New York. "We saw this huge spike, with a stealth-like nature this thing running wild very quickly, the case count skyrocketing," said Soto.

Fear was sparked, he said, "by the insidious nature of COVID, the speed and stealth with which it strikes. And we saw it very early on. Nobody knew how they were getting it. One moment you're in a social contact. The next moment, you were fighting for your life. And that bred a tremendous amount of anxiety in New Yorkers. We wanted to get out early and make sure that we were communicating to New Yorkers, *We're here for you. We're going to go through this with you. And we will get through this together.*"

Soto and colleagues had anticipated that in the early stages of the pandemic there would be widespread fear and uncertainty both within the ranks of the health system and among the public. People wondered how to protect themselves and their families. They wondered what the course of treatment was for those infected. They needed to know how the virus was transmitted.

"We went from this running start to this mission to fill the market with information," he said. "The creation process, the coordination process, and the distribution of that content [were] mammoth. We created over a thousand pieces of content and pushed that out in a very aggressive fashion" in an effort to "flood the market with reliable content" to combat fear and anxiety. Soto and colleagues created a campaign in one week focused on the theme that *Information is Healthy, Fear is Not.* The television commercial was a direct appeal for New Yorkers to call upon their native resilience. Soto wanted an authentic New York voice-over in the commercial and who better than actor Ray Romano? Not only did Romano have that distinctive New York accent, he had also grown up near Long Island Jewish Forest Hills Hospital in Queens. Generously, he volunteered to do the voice-over.

We New Yorkers have been through a lot.
But in our darkest moments
We always find the light . . .
We'll heal once again.
Together.
Because that's just what New Yorkers do.
Get the facts at northwell.edu/prepared and follow government guidance.

We believed that as a major source of care and a respected source of information in the medical realm, we had a responsibility to provide information and guidance every step of the way.

In addition to providing information through various communications channels, we also opened our doors to news organizations eager to report on what became the biggest story in the world. Terry Lynam, head of public relations, had built a valuable resource of knowledgeable clinicians and researchers who were also articulate and skilled communicators. Whatever the media request, Lynam had spokespersons available to explain the facts and tell the story fairly and eloquently in many cases. Various Northwell leaders appeared on all the major networks on such programs as the *TODAY Show*, *Face the Nation*, and *60 Minutes*, where five of our clinicians and one of us (Michael Dowling) were interviewed. After the *60 Minutes* segment the floodgates opened, and we were inundated with requests from media throughout the nation. Because we were at the epicenter of the outbreak and due to our willingness to open our doors to journalists seeking to report the story, there was significant media coverage of our work. Our doctors and nurses were interviewed for and quoted in articles in the *New York Times*, the *Wall Street Journal*, the *Washington Post*, *USA Today*, *Business Insider*, Bloomberg News, and other major daily newspapers, magazines, and wire services. We constructed a coronavirus digital resource center where we housed

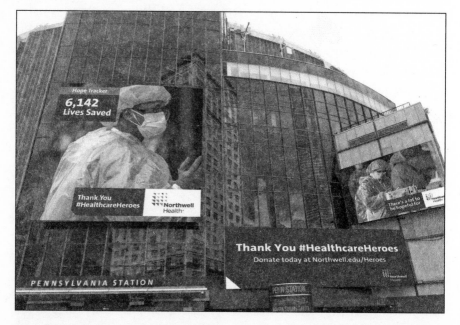

One of the many types of campaigns we ran during the crisis, giving hope to our patients.

consumer-friendly content designed to educate and inform. Nearly two million New Yorkers read the content. In the process, we were designated as Google's official source of COVID content for the Northeast.

Any discussion of the art of communication during the pandemic must include the masterful job Governor Andrew Cuomo did in articulating the reality on the ground. Cuomo's daily televised briefings were widely watched not only throughout New York but throughout the country. He excelled at making complex subjects simple and understandable. He stuck close to the data and, each day, showed charts indicating where the state was with respect to the peak. He was firm in his directives concerning isolation and social distancing, but, at the same time, his tone was comforting. Viewers felt they had a leader who was in command of the situation.

* * *

We communicated to many different audiences, including the Northwell Board of Trustees, to keep them up to date about the virus. We communicated internally to our employees so they would have the latest information about our latest developments, HR policies, testing, and more. We communicated within our emergency operations group on a near-constant basis with a minimum of two group virtual meetings per day. We used technology to foster communication between patients and their families. And on their own, nurses and doctors created team huddles to support and encourage one another. When clinicians stand in a circle, hold hands, and reflect or pray, they are reassuring one another that *yes, we can take this on and we will get through it together.* One of us, (Michael Dowling) was there at the front lines with the workers and by his mere presence communicated a powerful message of appreciation. One of the popular internal forms of communication among our frontline staff was a message written across their headbands stating: *Not today COVID.*

For many clinicians throughout the region the peak of the coronavirus was something of a blur. Doctors, nurses, and others worked themselves to exhaustion, often stunned by the lethal nature of the sickness around them. And it became clear to the communications team as New

York got past the peak that workers in health care were tired, frustrated, and, as they had been throughout, scared

"We wanted to fortify them, wanted to give them some resilience," said Soto. "And we started taking note of how a social movement was going on. New Yorkers were coming out and banging pots and pans, and the Fire Department was showing up and saluting these health-care heroes at 7 p.m. each night in New York. And we took that as a cue to create a new campaign" focused on expressing appreciation for the amazing work being done by frontline workers. The result was a campaign with television and radio commercials as well as print advertising with the theme: "To those who run toward the danger so we can stay safe: Thank you."

These nightly events were a powerful form of communication that bonded the people of New York with health-care workers. With the music, dancing, cheering, and banging of pots and pans, the people of the city—with one voice—were saying, *Thank you, bless you for what you are doing.* Nurses, doctors, and others were so moved by the display that it was not unusual to see them teary-eyed with gratitude as they entered the hospital for their overnight shift.

By early May, it was clear that the caseload was declining and there was a need to return to some semblance of normalcy. But that was complicated. Consumers were understandably concerned about how safe it would be to get treatment at a hospital where so many COVID patients had been. Many patients who needed nonurgent care—and even some who needed urgent care—were putting off going to the doctor's office or to the hospital because they believed it placed them at risk of getting infected. This presented a difficult communications challenge: to convince fearful people that our facilities were safe for them to return. This initiative started with communications to the six million people who have been patients in one of our facilities in recent years. We explained that our offices and hospitals were sterilized, that patients would be kept separate—no crowded waiting areas. We also noted that we had a long history of treating communicable disease safely within our offices and hospitals and knew well how to separate patients suspected of having a communicable disease from other patients.

Soto described the new world as "COVID in a chronic state. It's going to be here. Until there's a cure, it's here. So we have to make sure that consumers understand that the world is going to be different, that we're going to be able to treat you whether you have COVID or not." The situation presents an opportunity to engage with consumers in an effort to improve their health. "This has elevated the importance of health," said Soto. "There's this weird thing about health care. It's a low-interest category [with consumers] until you need it, then it becomes a high-interest category. And it has never been more important. It's front and center of the body politic."

He sees in this moment an opportunity to get consumers to think more deeply about their health and what they might do to improve their overall well-being by quitting smoking, losing some weight, or improving nutritional choices. "There's this really interesting opportunity to think about the preventative side of health . . . think about the journey of health, and think about the journey of wellness—and become a much more engaged partner with individuals through their life-long journey as your health needs or your family's needs change. Can Northwell have a much more prominent role in that relationship?"

* * *

As important as external communications were throughout the crisis, internal communications may have been even more important. Early on, our internal communications—emails, text messages, and video messages from one of us (Michael Dowling)—focused on instilling confidence that our incident command structure was preparing us well for the virus. We wanted to assure employees that we had learned from going through various emergencies in the past and that they were ready for this.

We communicated internally; for example, focusing on protocols for proper use of PPE, said Tom Sclafani, head of internal communications: "Our team members in the hospitals face communicable diseases each and every day, and so they are using PPE. But again, we wanted to just give a reminder to instill confidence that we would be relying on our training, relying on the protocols we had in place." Sclafani and his colleagues worked in partnership with clinical leaders to send out guidance on the proper uses of PPE, which mask to use under what conditions, how to preserve highly valuable N95 masks, when to change or get rid of PPE, and how to don and doff the equipment.

Another goal of internal communications was to advise staff of policy updates. Some policies changed multiple times over a few days, so Sclafani and his team had to get all of the communication regarding those changes out quickly. "Visitor protocols were changing at a certain point in March kind of on an almost daily basis, it seemed," he said. "First it was limited hours. Then it was limited number of people. Then shutting down all access to certain units, and then we reverted back because we felt like we probably were being too restrictive when it came to labor and delivery, for example. So that created a bit of an operational challenge. Then it created a bit of a communications challenge, which is just how quickly [you are] revising things, how quickly [you are] updating things." Sclafani set up a text message platform to send instant updates on policy changes, a rapid response channel that proved very successful in conveying information and boosting morale.

Sclafani said it was crucial to focus on sustaining morale and on caregiver well-being. "From a morale perspective," he said, "we know our clinical teams are exhausted. They're physically exhausted. They're probably emotionally drained. When you think about just the sheer volume of sick people, acutely sick people, that they have to care for and when you think about the number of mortalities related to this, it's really something that shakes people to their core and can really weaken them as they manage through this." That's why, with our internal communication as well as external, we wanted to recognize the frontline teams, celebrate success, and highlight the work of particular frontline nurses and doctors.

Among the work highlighted in our internal communications was that of Emily Fawcett, the registered nurse whose words form the Foreword to this book. At Lenox Hill Hospital, Emily worked with colleagues to create *hope huddles* where nurses shared success stories about patients surviving and going home to their families; stories that lifted morale and energized frontline teams.

One of the most moving events during the crisis came when Kelly McLaughlin, a nurse at Southside Hospital, organized an early morning event she called a Day of Hope. Our clinicians gathered outside the hospital, a thousand strong, nearly all donning a T-shirt with the Day of Hope message. It was one of those moments that reaffirmed our belief that, *yes, we will get through this. And, yes, we are made for this.*

CHAPTER TEN

Looking Forward— Preparing for the Future

The coronavirus is a painful reminder of life's fragility. Virtually overnight, it changed how we think about life and how we will live in the future. The severity and speed of the virus presented a test for which no one in the world of health care was fully prepared. Yet, overall, the medical community in the epicenter that was New York responded to the crisis with grit, determination, and much success. The pandemic revealed the professionalism and commitment of health-care workers throughout the country, particularly in New York, where we were inundated and nearly overwhelmed. But a sturdy partnership with Governor Cuomo and hospital leaders and workers got us through it all. The crisis revealed uplifting public appreciation for clinicians and all staff. People cheering in the streets and delivering food and supplies to hospitals had clinicians in tears of joy and appreciation. There was a new cooperative spirit among competitors. The hospitals and health systems in New York have not always been known for their cooperative ventures, but the coronavirus changed that. We all did what we could to lift one another up—sharing ambulances, doctors, oxygen supplies, PPE, and ventilators. This knitting together of resources and capabilities is a must going forward. The governor has issued a call to action insisting that all of us in the health-care community continue to serve the people in whatever way we can during emergencies, and to do it together.

One thing that health-care workers did together was stand up to fear.

In the crossfire hurricane that was the coronavirus pandemic, fear was always there; day shift, night shift, it didn't matter. The doctors and nurses, respiratory therapists and others—these men and women who carried our health system on their shoulders—were "surrounded by fear twenty-four hours a day," in the words of Northwell Chief Nursing Executive Maureen White. She walked the wards checking in with staff, listening, encouraging, and she kept hearing about the fear. "Even when they were sleeping, they were telling me how it was never a quiet sleep; it was always restless, always the fears, always the worries about, *what if?* When they were here, they were thinking about their family members at home, and when they were home, they were thinking about their patients and their teammates back at the hospital and wanting to go back to help. When I was on rounds they told me [that] the first week was overwhelming. We didn't know what was coming at us; there was no playbook for caring for these types of patients. This was not the flu that everybody had been saying prior to that point. This was something very different." They were seeing more sickness and death than they had ever witnessed and they did not want that to be their fate, or the fate of their children, spouse, or parents.

These frontline workers were baptized amid the crisis into a new world; strange, forbidding, isolating, and exhausting. There were no blueprints for how to handle it, but medical workers kept showing up for their shifts even as patients died, even as colleagues died. And it was by understanding the depth of the fear that we learned a great lesson: that the men and women who have chosen health care as a career will take on any challenge, overcome any obstacle, to do the majestic work of caring for their fellow human beings. We knew it in a way before the coronavirus, but this horrific event put their oaths to the most rigorous test: Risk your own life and maybe the lives of your loved ones to help another human being.

Rx: Thirteen Steps to Prepare for Current and Future Viral Threats

In this chapter we outline the significant changes needed to prepare for the current and future viral threats. Whether the coronavirus breaks out this fall, winter, or next spring, we need to be prepared. And we must be doubly prepared for what lies beyond that with the potential of a virus even more lethal than this one. We believe that these thirteen prescriptive steps, if taken seriously, will save lives. On their own, these actions are powerful; taken together they have the potential to transform our collective ability to fight future pandemics.

1. Plan ahead.
2. Build an emergency management culture.
3. Commit to regulatory flexibility.
4. Urgently address inequities in access to care.
5. Protect the physical and emotional health of staff.
6. Recognize the benefits of integrated health systems in a crisis.
7. Partner with government, other health systems, and community groups.
8. Reverse America's cultural disrespect for science.
9. Develop leadership at every level of the organization.
10. Accelerate the movement to virtual care.
11. Educate the public.
12. Increase focus on safety measures in congregate settings.
13. Commit to creating a New Normal.

1. Plan ahead.

Failing to plan ahead risks the possibility of falling behind the speed of the virus, and if you fall behind, you may never catch up. You cannot put something together on the fly when you're in a situation like the COVID crisis. You cannot start from behind and run fast enough to catch up to the speed of viral spread. The most obvious and most important step toward preparing for next time is to apply the lessons learned during the COVID-19 pandemic *now* while they are fresh in our collective psyche. Even as we work to reopen our system to care for the pent-up demand for services that built during the crisis, we are simultaneously preparing for the next COVID wave. In 2020 our nation was caught off guard and scrambled to catch up to the virus. The responsibility to plan ahead falls to the government, of course, but also to every hospital and health system in the country. To do anything less than prepare in an aggressive fashion now, given what we have been through, would be negligent. Planning ahead means planning for *the worst*. With increasing urbanization in China, India, and elsewhere, human beings and animals inevitably come into closer contact, making transmission of a virus from animals to humans more likely. In recent decades, hundreds of new infectious diseases have emerged.

Observed Dr. Kevin Tracey:

> There will be another emerging disease with the potential to do even more damage than this coronavirus did. If the coronavirus was a seventy-five-year flood, we need to be prepared for the thousand-year flood. The Army Corps of Engineers had a goal of preparing New Orleans for a hundred-year flood, and then they built dams and dikes for a twenty-year flood. Holland, on the other hand, prepared for a hundred-year flood and then built dikes for a thousand-year flood. And the differences are stark. A hurricane comes into New Orleans and it floods the city and people die. And Holland is bone dry for many, many years. I think we have to be thinking about preparing for the thousand-year event because there are lots of viruses that are ten or a hundred times more lethal than the flu, and that's what we have to worry about. Because when you scale those numbers, you're talking not about one or two hundred thousand Americans dying. You're talking about tens of millions of Americans dying in six months.

What is history's great lesson about catastrophic viruses? They keep coming back. "It's undeniable that this will happen again," continued Tracey.

> Saying it wouldn't happen again is like saying we're never going to have another hurricane or another tornado or another flood. We will have more serious weather problems and we will have more pandemics. You prepare by having better processes in place for more rapid isolation of the virus and more rapid identification and isolation of infected hosts. For instance, why didn't Ebola spread much more far and wide than it did?

Because of effective clamping down on identification of cases and isolation. And we learned from this event that all the draconian measures we put in place with closing things down and social distancing did flatten the curve. We learned from this event that you can intervene as a society, as a nation, as a state, and you can save lives and you can change the behavior of the spread. But if it happens with a virus that's much more lethal, we're going to have to do it much better and much faster.

Essential to proper planning ahead is addressing the dangerous flaws in the medical supply chain. It is painfully obvious that in the United States we have to be ready in the future to test for infection and to provide the protective equipment our clinicians depend upon. And we should never again have less than a robust stockpile of ventilators and other essential equipment. To achieve these goals we cannot rely solely on any one nation to fill these needs. Overreliance on China to manufacture vital supplies is a perilous gamble. There is no question that domestic manufacturing of some items is essential and toward that end, we at Northwell are considering acquiring a supply company to achieve a measure of self-sufficiency when it comes to vital supplies. Domestic manufacturing costs are a good deal steeper than overseas costs. So be it. Having a reliable domestic manufacturing capability for PPE and other essentials is more than worth it. Stockpiles awaiting an emergency will grow within health systems as well as state and federal warehouses. If we as a country are smart, we will also figure out a way to avoid the insane bidding war for necessary supplies and equipment that pit one health system and state against everyone else and the federal government to boot. An important lesson from the coronavirus was the shocking inadequacy of our ability to test for the virus. Preparation for the future must include a capability to test quickly and widely across large populations.

Another form of overreliance involves the manufacturing concentration of pharmaceuticals in China and India. In the United States, we have to establish domestic manufacturing facilities for lifeline medications. "The United States Army didn't outsource its bullet-making to China," said Dr. Kevin Tracey. "The Army makes its own bullets. And we should be making our own drugs, or at least have a mechanism to make drugs in an emergency. The United States as a nation has an obligation to restore some essential manufacturing capabilities on our own shores because if the virus had killed and disabled more people in Asia, we wouldn't have had any drugs."

A key part of our preparation had come when we had taken the time and effort to convert dozens of units into negative pressure rooms to protect patients and staff.

2. Build an emergency management culture.

The virus exposed a major weakness in American health care that must be addressed if health systems are going to be ready for the next pandemic. This is an enormous task and we as a country ignore it at our peril. We have mentioned culture numerous times through this book for a very good reason: It is the foundational element upon which a competent emergency response system is constructed. It involves an organizational belief in the efficacy of an emergency capability as well as respect for the process of building an emergency operations team, training that team, funding that team, and assuring that the team trains regularly in anticipation of a crisis. Gene Tangney, a top Northwell executive, talked about the "muscle memory" training builds. How do you know when an organization is imbued with an emergency management culture? When the organization is "comfortable being uncomfortable in a crisis." An emergency culture in a hospital or health system means more awareness, better preparation, and more professional execution.

This culture starts at the top of the organization. What message does it convey to clinicians literally risking their lives on the front line when senior leaders are not visible and not supporting them? In contrast, within our organization, senior leadership joined our teams at the front throughout. One of the key attributes of our health system is our spirit of a team culture. "I would argue that team mentality and inclusive leadership culture are the foundation of our health system success," said Tangney. "We faced many disasters in the past that were successfully managed by a strong incident command structure," where the team members worked in a respectful, friendly way. The team members get along well. We have disagreements, but those are typically solved quickly and amicably.

An important aspect of preparing for a pandemic involves creating a robust early warning system for clinicians, hospitals, and public health officials to receive alerts about atypical spikes in patients seeking care in ambulatory sites and emergency departments. This early-warning system allows for rapid responses based on up-to-the-minute data from a variety of sources both public and private.

3. Commit to regulatory flexibility.

It would be profoundly regrettable if governments at all levels reverted to the same sets of rules, laws, and regulations governing health systems that were waived or suspended during the crisis. Among the most important lessons of our experience in this pandemic is that regulatory flexibility promotes speed, creativity, and efficiency—and saves lives. When the Centers for Medicare and Medicaid Services, the Food and Drug Administration, and state regulatory agencies waived rules, they demonstrated the potential for a new age of innovation in health care. Hospitals and health systems demonstrated that we can act faster and more effectively when freed from the constraints of regulatory micromanagement. We had the freedom to put beds where we had never before had beds; to create an ICU capacity we had never imagined; and to create new machinery that helped people breathe!

The pandemic was a time of sickness and death, but it was also a time of innovation which, in health care, has too often been a cumbersome process. Throughout the medical world there are entrenched interests with the power to thwart change. Chairs of medical departments, experienced physicians who are comfortable doing things *their way*, and administrators wary of a loss of authority are often resistant to change. People in a particular department may be prone to constructing a silo around their turf, but the advantage of a crisis is that the silos fall away and the normal rules do not apply. Under the incident command structure, leaders are empowered to make major changes on the spot. We did a lot of that during the pandemic and learned that it worked to our benefit. Did we step on toes? Absolutely. Break down bureaucratic barriers? Yes. The result: We did things in days that under normal conditions would have taken months. For example, our scientists, in a matter of days, used 3D-printed parts to adapt machines used on patients with sleep apnea into machines that served as backup ventilators, which was lifesaving. When the dust settled we saw that the speed of innovation did not sacrifice quality and stability. In the future, there will be no excuses for lumbering innovation.

The question now is: to what extent do we revert to a prior regulatory norm? Governor Cuomo's decision to waive scores of regulations—such as the prohibition on doctors from other states practicing in New York—gave us the manpower and freedom to care for patients in the best possible ways. Job number one, as we coordinate our efforts with other hospitals and health systems as well as with the government, is to make sure that many of these regulations are retired while others are modified. When we examined the rules and laws regulating our industry, it was striking that implicit in many was a basic mistrust of health-care workers. It is not that we do not believe in regulation. We certainly do. As we've stated, a number of our senior leaders at Northwell once held top regulatory positions in the state government. But times have changed. Many rules and regulations have not aged well. We believe that the presumption should tilt a bit more in the direction that health-care workers can be relied upon to do the right thing for their patients. If that presumption cannot be made and codified after what we have just been through, then nothing will convince regulators of doctors and nurses' commitment to the finest care for their patients.

4. Urgently address inequities in access to care.

Poorer communities in New York and elsewhere were disproportionately harmed by the virus. It is incumbent upon all of us in health care to work with the government as well as civic and community groups and churches to take the steps needed to increase health overall in these communities so they have a greater degree of protection the next time a virus arrives. If we work with these communities now we can make them more resilient next time. The greater likelihood that poor people as well as people from minority populations will die from the virus presents further evidence of a health divide within American society. Health-care organizations such as ours, working in partnership with government and social service agencies, need to make a more determined effort to work on preventive care in underserved areas. This includes tackling the social determinants of health. Certainly, greater efforts at prevention could make a difference. Complicating factors making people more vulnerable to COVID include high blood pressure and obesity that people living in poverty are more likely to develop. Chronic diseases that plague minority neighborhoods must be addressed by the combined efforts of public and private health systems along with the government and community organizations. The task for the near-term future is for health systems working with the state to target new ways of addressing the social determinants of health that contribute to the disparities.

In New York, Governor Cuomo has identified this as a major priority. The efforts of major hospitals and health systems in this area have lacked coordination in the past. A stronger partnership among provider groups and with the state offers new possibilities for progress. We demonstrated this in the spring of 2020 when we worked cooperatively with the governor's office and the New York State Department of Health to offer antibody and diagnostic testing in Black and Latino communities working through local churches. Also, physician leaders at Northwell collaborated with faculty at the State University of New York at Albany to study the impact of COVID on minority communities throughout the state.

As we look ahead, there seems little doubt that hospitals, ambulatory sites, and physicians in underserved areas in New York will need a greater investment for both capital improvements and operating costs going forward. Many of these facilities are under financial stress and need help. We owe the people who use them a better experience; we owe the people who work in them an updated environment. As a society we owe the hospitals, ambulatory sites, and the providers who work in these areas the quality facilities and financial stability necessary to improving the delivery of care. The disparities in outcomes based on race and income during the COVID crisis should also accelerate discussion about the best way to provide the universal health coverage that every American deserves as a fundamental human right.

5. Protect the physical and emotional health of staff.
PPE protects staff members physically and emotionally and boosts morale. With the right PPE, staff members could do their jobs knowing they were being protected. It is estimated that approximately 14 percent

of the New York state population was infected with the virus, with large numbers asymptomatic. Given the proximity of frontline workers to many patients with the virus, you would think they would be infected at a much higher rate than the general population. But we found through testing that our workers were infected at a rate comparable to the general population—an indication of how protective PPE turned out to be. This evidence gives our teams a high degree of confidence that, with the proper protective gear, they can confront the challenges of an infectious environment in the future with very good chances of remaining healthy.

Much of the focus during the crisis was on PPE, beds, and ventilators, but *the* essential asset was staff, and we did everything we could to protect staff physically and emotionally. We scoured the world for additional N95 masks. We paid for hotel rooms for staff members not wanting to go home and potentially infect a family member. We set up *tranquility tents* to provide frontline staff with time and space to reflect, meditate, or pray. We provided counselors on-site to help people get through their grief, anxiety, and sadness. We initiated a healing and recovery process focused on addressing the physical, psychological, and spiritual impacts of the crisis on our workers. We will continue to watch staff very closely for some time to come, looking for signs of psychological stress, so that we can provide whatever help they need. At Northwell, we faced staggering financial losses totaling $1.6 billion, but as the crisis began to wind down we made a decision to pay bonuses to fifty thousand employees, and in addition to the bonuses, we also gave staff members an additional week of paid vacation. Why did we do it in the face of such historic losses? *Because we had to show our people in every way possible how valuable they are;* how much we appreciate their efforts every day, how much we valued their courage and professionalism in the most difficult time our health system has ever faced. These doctors, nurses, respiratory therapists, techs, housekeepers, transport workers—these people are the lifeblood of our organization. We need them to know how deeply they are appreciated as we move ahead in uncertain times when they will be called upon, at some point, to reprise their heroic roles. And we are always mindful of the fact that we know from the data that there is a direct correlation between satisfied employees and satisfied patients.

In pursuit of adequate staff in an emergency, we are creating a medical reserve corps within Northwell. This involves enlisting nurses and doctors who have retired in the last three years and who would be interested in being available to us in times of crisis. We will conduct regular training to keep them competent in their fields, and create a database that tells us exactly who is available with the skills we require for whatever the emergency happens to be.

6. Recognize the benefits of integrated health systems in a crisis.

For some years now consolidation has been criticized by academics and others who argue that mergers of hospital systems typically result in higher prices and no better quality or even a decline in quality. And it is true that there have been numerous mergers that have not lived up to their potential. Consumers have a right to demand better performance from large integrated systems, and we think the performance of systems like ours during the crisis will cause a reassessment of their value. Dr. Ira S. Nash, executive director of Northwell Health Physician Partners, wrote in *Modern Healthcare* that:

> The conventional explanation is that hospitals and doctors are seeking more economic power. Size, the argument goes, allows health systems to demand higher reimbursement rates from commercial payers, which have themselves merged into a handful of enormous national carriers. Several recent studies contend that provider consolidation, often undertaken under the banner of improved efficiency and quality, may raise the cost of care in local markets, without apparent improvements in patient outcomes. But there is more to the story.
>
> What the simple narrative doesn't capture is the changing nature of clinical medicine. Hospitals are no longer places where patients get admitted electively for diagnostic testing or spend days or weeks recovering from surgery or an acute medical illness. Even before the COVID-19 pandemic, they were places filled with patients too sick to be anywhere else. Contemporary hospital care is labor intensive, know-how intensive, technology intensive and capital intensive; high

quality inpatient care now requires organizational scale to
assemble and manage these resources.[*]

It is true that hospitals are expensive to build and maintain. It is true
that it is often more cost-effective to manage patients in outpatient settings, and there is no doubt that health care is moving inexorably in the
direction of providing care in locations as close to the patient's home as
possible. In the years to come, in fact, more and more care will be delivered in the home, much of it through virtual interactions between doctor
and patient. This is a very positive development, and at Northwell we are
moving aggressively in this direction. But as the Marines like to say: In
a ground war, when you need a tank, *only a tank will do.* So, too, in a
global pandemic, when you need an integrated hospital system, *only an
integrated hospital system will do.*

And the capability within a system to distribute patients, supplies,
and staff exactly where they are needed is lifesaving. The intricacy of
load balancing is not immediately obvious, but it was among the most
challenging aspects of our work—especially early on when our hospitals
in Forest Hills and Valley Stream were inundated. We were able to relieve
the pressure in both locations by safely moving hundreds of patients to
other locations, all within our own system. That is a benefit of having
an integrated twenty-three-hospital system. But not everyone has such a
system. There are many smaller stand-alone entities that are highly capable of caring for their patients in normal times but are stressed during an
emergency. The solution is to create an integrated load-balancing system
among all hospitals, whether they are part of the same entity or not.
Some of this happened on the fly during the COVID period, but it was
more haphazard than not and too many hospitals, especially public facilities, did not have a partner to serve as a relief valve. It is our obligation
as health-care leaders to construct an emergency network throughout
New York and beyond that leaves no one out; that ensures that every
hospital and system in an emergency shares capabilities and resources so

---

[*] Dr. Ira Nash, "Big Challenges Require Large-scale Solutions—As the COVID-19 Pandemic Is Proving," *Modern Healthcare*, April 2020.

that never again will patients, disproportionately in poor neighborhoods, suffer from a lack of care.

7. Partner with government, other health systems, and community groups.

This experience revealed the need for more partnerships among a variety of organizations including local government agencies, civic groups, law enforcement, businesses, and religious organizations. In a crisis, the various component parts of networks can work together to educate and encourage people to follow medical recommendations. We emerge from the crisis with a renewed determination at Northwell to actively build more partnerships not only to prepare for a crisis, per se, but to facilitate greater educational and prevention efforts to improve the overall wellness of communities at the granular level. Networks also allow for shared sacrifice in an emergency. Some areas of New York were slammed by the virus while others were largely unaffected. In a crisis, resources from unaffected areas can be used to support communities under greater stress from infections. We are determined to solidify these types of relationships now, before the next crisis. This will enable us to coordinate with local government agencies and departments that were not always in sync this time, creating confusion for the people actually doing the work.

By their very nature, epidemics tend to move from one location to another, peaking at different times in different geographical areas. This was certainly the case with the coronavirus. While in New York we were inundated with sickness, many other parts of the country were relatively unharmed when we were at our peak. But by the start of summer the virus was raging in other parts of the country, including Texas, California, Arizona, and elsewhere. Given this pattern, Northwell physician Dr. Lawrence Smith suggested that we—and others—partner not only with community groups in our area, but with health systems in other parts of the state and other parts of the country. "We needed to have partners who were far away from us," he said, "and when we were overwhelmed, they would send us teams of people to help us out, and then inevitably we would get better and they would get overwhelmed and we would reciprocate and send teams to them. I think in the future we will have those partners all lined up." An example of this sort of help during the coronavirus pandemic came when Intermountain Health in Utah sent a team of clinicians to New York to help us. In addition, a team from the University of Rochester came to our system to help. We are eternally grateful to both organizations.

8. Reverse America's cultural disrespect for science.

Underlying the coronavirus assault on America is a problem so foundational and so disturbing that it is difficult to imagine our society solving the issue in anything less than a generation; namely, ignorance of and lack of respect for science. It goes down to the grass roots where the anti-vaccination movement has gained traction promoting willful ignorance. The attitude is that the scientists are not telling the truth about vaccinations, climate change, etc. It is people who know nothing about science, yet who feel entitled to make judgments about scientific issues. For issues such as climate change and vaccinations to have become so politicized suggests to Dr. Kevin Tracey that "many people in today's society do not understand science or care about it." Part of the problem, he said, is that the essential nature of scientific research is the antithesis of what is today most celebrated in American life:

> The materialistic culture of the United States celebrates money and it celebrates instant fame. But successful scientists work on projects for many, many years at low pay and out of the limelight. Many young people today are turned off by the concept of long-time horizons to success. History has shown that the persistent and consistent approach to science cures diseases and eradicates viruses. We can only hope that this current crisis will elevate some scientists, like [Dr. Anthony Fauci], to a well-deserved hero status, and will attract more young people to become like him.

Tracey worries that political and government leaders might not make the necessary commitments to science and research that are warranted. "It can't be that we now rush back to business as usual," he said.

The genius of John F. Kennedy's "to the moon and back" speech was that it created a ten-year process of continued investment and growth. It wasn't that Sputnik happened and then DARPA was created, and then NASA was created, and then there was a space race. It was sustained investments over decades. And that's what we have to do now. We need to do a ten-year march of preparation for this because it will come again. And next time it could be worse. As part of that, we need to increase our investments in public health and in research because research will not only provide the answer for the current coronavirus, but is essential to the discovery of yet unknown therapies. But you can't start investing in research after the problem starts. There has to be a sustained investment in the infrastructure so that the people are in place and the laboratories are in place. And then the solutions will come faster.

Increased investments in the NIH, CDC, and other entities have the potential to pay great dividends when it comes to protecting our nation from future pandemics.

The United States needs a greater ability to start clinical trials quickly. There is nothing like a crisis to break down barriers and smash through bureaucratic rules. In a medical emergency we demonstrated that we have the ability to set up rigorous scientific clinical trials in a matter of days. This would have been unheard of prior to the coronavirus. But now that we have that ability, we will put it to good use in the future.

9. Allow leadership to flourish at every level of your organization.

Leadership at all levels of an organization is about telling the truth, building trust, developing a sense of community, and being willing to be held accountable. As we reflect upon the crisis in New York, it seems clear that leadership was the glue that held us all together. There was the leadership of Governor Andrew Cuomo, getting up in front of the cameras every day, reporting the data and the situation with full transparency, making the tough decisions to protect the public, unwilling to hide behind sentiment or opinion and instead letting science and facts lead the way. Our system followed the governor's lead in laying out the facts as we found them—no obfuscation, no twist in one political direction or another. We sought to portray confidence and optimism throughout the crisis with the goal of informing the public as a means of calming fears.

There were our C-suite leaders out on the front lines day after day, being present with the frontline troops, showing them that the entire health system stood with them. There was the leadership of people on the front lines; the people in our organization promoting programs that enabled frontline workers to deal with their fears and anxieties; the nurse leaders who learned to build morale by celebrating every patient who made it through the nightmare; the nurse and physician executives who spent time talking, listening, and encouraging staff on the front lines, making clear that we had their backs. There were thousands of examples. We had leaders who volunteered for some of the toughest and most dangerous assignments. We had a cadre of physician leaders who did the heroic work of recalculating best practices practically by the hour as we learned about the virus. There were leaders of our incident command team calmly transitioning the team to the largely unknown world of Microsoft Teams. And our clinical and administrative teams on that terrible night when Forest Hills was nearly overrun—that was one of the best examples of leadership you will ever see. Doctors and nurses taking time to talk to console the family of a dying patient—going on FaceTime—to share the final moments of a loved one's life—that was so difficult and heartbreaking and it, too, was leadership. In the future, organizations that have respected leaders marbled throughout every level of an organization will respond much more effectively to crisis than those that have failed to develop such a cadre of leaders.

10. Accelerate the movement to virtual care.
The COVID crisis was an unfortunate but nonetheless remarkable opportunity to spread the use of telehealth in the United States beyond what would have seemed possible just months earlier. Telehealth is a fantastic way for patients in need of care to gain access with a tool—a smartphone—that is already an integral part of their lives. In addition to providing patients access to their doctors, it also provides a portal to connect with a nurse practitioner, a nutritionist, a psychotherapist, a lactation consultant—the full panoply of medical specialties.

The breakthrough for telehealth came during the COVID crisis when the Centers for Medicare and Medicaid Services (CMS) announced that it would reimburse doctors at the same rate whether the visit was in person or virtual. Telehealth was never financially viable before because insurers paid a fraction of in-person visit rates for virtual visits. With comparable rates for in-person and virtual visits, telehealth can be financially viable for doctors.

The advantages of telehealth are numerous. Such visits allow doctors—even those in quarantine—to treat from the home, office, or wherever else they happen to be, noted Dr. Martin Doerfler, senior vice president for clinical strategy and development. For patients, there are no worries about traffic, parking, or going out into an environment where you might be exposed to the virus. Stay home, safe, and comfortable— and get the full attention and expertise of your doctor in the comfort of your home. This is especially valuable for patients who feel very sick.

Before the crisis, the use of telehealth by our physicians was at only a modest level, but when the crisis struck, telehealth use spiked in a way we have never before experienced. "We got lucky," said Doerfler. "We were preparing for a change in the telehealth landscape and our preparations were fairly mature when this happened, and we were able to scale incredibly quickly on what we had. On February 28, we were averaging about 150 visits a month on our telehealth platform called American Well. On May 2, we had 3500 and on May 4, we had 6400."

The recent common expression about telehealth has become: *The genie is out of the bottle and not going back.* But unless the genie is paid to be out of the bottle there will be a problem with the spread of telehealth. It is very good news that Medicare has agreed to pay the same rate for virtual as for in-person visits. Will they sustain that policy? The signs are positive but there is not yet a guarantee. Typically, commercial insurance companies follow their lead. But will they do so with telehealth? "That's the hundred-thousand-dollar question," said Alexandra Trinkoff, deputy general counsel at Northwell. "I can tell from the pushback that we're getting from managed care plans that they recognize that members are going to want to continue getting care through telehealth. However, they're very nervous that this increased access to care is going to increase the number of visits required for a patient and really drive health insurance costs up, because it could provide almost too much utilization, too much access."

Howard Gold, Northwell executive vice president and chief of managed care, is wary of commercial insurers when it comes to telehealth reimbursements. "It's still a fight on telehealth," he said. "That has become a new frontline issue and [the insurers are] making all kinds of distinctions: *Is it a telephone call, is it a video, is it a conference call?* How do we make distinctions? And I said, 'Look, my point of view is that a doctor's time is a doctor's time, and we should be paid for that time.'"

Dr. Lawrence Smith agrees. "Telehealth will never permanently catch on if you don't get paid at the exact same rate as non-telehealth," he said. "Your time is worth your time. If telehealth makes your time worth half of what it used to be, no one will do it."

11. Educate the public.

One of the essential ways to deal with a pandemic is prevention and to prevent spread the cooperation of the public is essential. Effective prevention allows health systems such as ours to deal with manageable numbers of sick patients. Without effective prevention, health-care providers can be overwhelmed.

People in New York for the most part did a creditable job at prevention by following public health guidelines. It is inconvenient and frustrating to follow guidelines but it is absolutely critical to continue the preventive effort and not to let our guard down. We have seen the consequences across the US South and Southwest.

In many parts of the country Americans followed the advice of public health experts and elected officials. In New York, for example, Governor Cuomo stuck to science and millions of New Yorkers did the things that controlled the virus. They quarantined, wore masks, followed social distancing, avoided large gatherings, etc. Consistency in messaging from leaders makes a difference. The recommendations of the leading physicians and scientists in New York were perfectly aligned with messages from the governor.

Would things have been different nationally had the president been similarly aligned with the country's leading medical experts? What would leadership look like from the president? It would have been Mr. Trump asking the nation to follow the science and pledging that he would do exactly that. How difficult would it have been for the president to stand up and say *I agree with Drs. Fauci and Birx and I am going to follow the guidelines of wearing a mask, social distancing where possible, etc., and I hope you, the American people, will join me in doing the same.*

When the president strikes a discordant note, however, the public is confused. Mixed signals from leaders such as the president and some governors mean less prevention, greater spread. By minimizing the nature of the threat, it is likely that some Americans let down their guard and, consistent with the president's messages, failed to take the pandemic seriously. While we were fortunate to have strong scientific leaders at the national level throughout the crisis, the same cannot be said of the nation's top elected official. Leadership requires a commitment to understanding reality and the courage to bring that reality to the people. President Trump fell short of any reasonable standard of leadership throughout. The president's claims about the efficacy of various drugs, in the absence of scientific proof, disrupted serious scientific research. His unwillingness to wear a mask sent a divisive signal to his followers. Who would have believed that the wearing of a mask during a viral pandemic could be seen as anything other than common sense? Had the president acted more responsibly and more in line with data and science, how many American lives could have been saved? The moral burden of having to answer that question is haunting. At Northwell, our teams fought the virus at every turn. It would have helped to have the leader of our country fighting alongside.

12. Increase focus on safety measures in congregate settings.

It is sound public policy to close down crowded gatherings such as movie theaters, Broadway shows, houses of worship, sports venues, etc. Such congregate settings are a petri dish for the spread of virus. Some congregate living locations cannot be closed down, however. Nursing homes, group homes, and assisted-living facilities play an integral role in the continuum of care for patients who are older, more vulnerable, and in need of constant care and attention. All of us in health care and government must work together to improve the care and safety of individuals in these settings. These facilities require a comprehensive and laser-focused approach dealing with infection-control practices, the availability of PPE, the training and education of staff, appropriate testing as well as an ongoing review of visitation policies and admission criteria. As evidence clearly demonstrated during this crisis, people in these crowded settings are at much higher risk of getting ill and dying. The percentage of total deaths in nursing homes was as high as 77 percent in states such as Rhode Island and Minnesota. Internationally it was a similar story. In Canada the percentage of deaths in long-term-care facilities reached 81 percent, followed by Ireland at 62 percent, France at 51 percent, and Sweden at 49 percent. New York, at 21 percent, ranked among the five best states in the nation in this category. Nonetheless, there was too much death in these facilities and we have work to do to prepare safer congregate environments going forward.

13. Commit to creating a New Normal.

We are not going back to normal. There is no going back. The only normal will be new and we must embrace it to be ready for the next time. Our experience with COVID changed the world. In health care, it forces organizations such as Northwell to find new ways of doing our work. What will health care look like in the years to come? We know that telehealth is an important part of the future. We know that getting care delivery as close to the home as possible is a goal. But what else? It is our job now to try and see over the horizon and to adapt to that future in ways that provide greater health-care equity, quality, and value than ever before. We are forced to do this due to a catastrophic event. At the same time, we welcome the opportunity to find the best pathways forward. We must not let the lessons go to waste. For example, we are in the process of reconstructing Lenox Hill Hospital on Manhattan's Upper East Side. How should we rethink what that facility should look like in light of COVID? What capabilities should be built in that we had not previously considered? We must rethink everything so that we create the most dynamic New Normal possible.

Essential to the New Normal is emergency management preparation. In the new normal we will examine old ways of doing business and adapt them to the future. We all have to create a new relationship with consumers, building trust and working with patients on new ways to access treatment and engage with our health-care professionals. We need to rethink how we deliver care and where we deliver care and how we work more assertively to keep people healthy. Perhaps we can work more aggressively to use telehealth in a concerted effort to partner with patients—including many in underserved areas—on their journey toward a more healthful lifestyle. At Northwell, because we were out front on the pandemic, we have built additional trust with our communities, and we fully intend to use that trust to educate people more broadly and deeply about their overall health and well-being. We have their attention as never before and we want to help them develop healthier habits.

In the new normal our reach will be broader into the community, as we work with a variety of businesses hungry for guidance about medical best practices for reopening, as well as for testing. We believe the future is bright. We as an organization got through the worst health crisis in a century pretty well. But we will do better next time because we are taking seriously the lessons enunciated in this book and summarized in this chapter. We hope other health systems in other parts of the country take note of some of these hard earned lessons. Governments, too. Because preparing the right way for next time could save countless lives.

APPENDIX I

Voices from the Front

Ross Feinman is a registered nurse in LIJ Medical Center's emergency department. He is also a professional paramedic.

I've been an emergency department nurse for more than eight years, including the last four at LIJ (Long Island Jewish) Medical Center. Right now, we are dubbing LIJ as "COVID city" because it is the center of this pandemic.

When I arrive for my shift at 7:30 a.m., the ambulance bay is empty. All patients are inside. It's quiet . . . for now.

We have a team member screening all patients outside the emergency department. It's very important to screen them so we don't mix COVID-positive patients with those who aren't sick with the virus. We have a responsibility to our patients to keep them safe.

Inside the hospital, the constant calls overhead for medical response are accelerating. We hear them every ten to thirty minutes. Patients are crashing to floors, needing air and breathing tubes. Some of them are no longer with us.

Taking care of COVID-positive patients has been a challenge. We provide chest therapy, an airway clearance technique to drain the lungs. We have also been proning patients, which means turning them to lay on their bellies. This helps them breathe easier and has saved a lot of patients from being intubated.

At LIJ, patient overflow has crept into the emergency department of Cohen Children's Medical Center. That's how packed we are. Taking a look back outside at our ambulance bay, there are no more available parking spaces, each filled with a Northwell ambulance and some are from out-of-state, FEMA-activated ambulances. One is from Chicago.

Big thanks to them. We need them.

LIJ Medical Center has a beautiful lobby, like a resort or hotel. But you wouldn't know it right now. I used to take breaks on one of the calming sides of the lobby, but they are using it for COVID patient overflow.

As much as we want to say we are trained for this, we are not. We are not trained for a pandemic. We are not trained for people quarantining. We are not trained for social distancing. The problem is, we can't send people home fast enough. And we don't have space to bring people upstairs.

Regardless of these challenges, everyone—doctors, nurses, environmental workers, and many more—at the hospital has stepped up. The community has stepped up, bringing supplies and food. We are all working together to take care of as many people as possible. While it may seem as if it will get worse before it gets better, I tell myself, every day we are a shift closer to it ending.

Later around 8:30 p.m., my shift is over. I walk to my car after a thirteen-hour day. You can see marks on my face from peeling off my N95 mask.

Nicole Fishman, RN, is a nurse manager at Huntington Hospital.
During the COVID-19 crisis, there's been an even greater focus on caring for our patients as whole people in light of very limited visitation policies. They sometimes get scared having minimal contact with their friends and families. But my staff and I have been proactively calling family members and giving them updates on their loved one throughout the day. We are also using iPads and tablets to FaceTime and Skype with families, so they can share their love with our patients.

When we are communicating with families through tablets, I think about my own parents and how I would want them to be treated if they were in this situation.

It's been amazing getting so much support from throughout our hospital. All of the people we're caring for are either suspected or confirmed

COVID-19 patients. So everyone is isolated and requires a higher level of care. We are managing this by working as a team, staying strong, and supporting each other in any way that we can. As expected, we're taking everything day by day.

Wearing all of this additional gear can make it harder to breathe, which is why we need more frequent breaks. I try to take advantage of any time away, going outside for fresh air and to clear my head.

All of Huntington Hospital's employees have been so appreciative of the meals that we've received from community donations. It's been very helpful to not have to worry about cooking or preparing food. We can focus on what matters most—our patients.

One thing I've been surprised about is that younger patients—people in their forties, fifties, and sixties—are deteriorating faster than I would have anticipated. Some don't have a past medical history of preexisting conditions.

I'm fortunate to have a very supportive boyfriend who's at home cooking and taking care of things while I'm out fighting COVID-19. Many of the other nurses on my unit have supportive significant others who have been writing encouraging letters and packing food for us.

When I leave work, I take several precautions in an attempt to protect my boyfriend from this dangerous virus. I change my shoes before I get into the car and shower immediately when I get home. I take all of my clothes off right by the door and throw them straight into the washing machine on a hot water setting. I feel safer being on my unit versus out in the community because we're all wearing the proper protective gear and the unit is constantly being cleaned.

Elyse Isopo is a nurse practitioner in North Shore University Hospital's Intensive Care Unit.
Every morning and every night, I take my temperature to make sure I am healthy enough to take care of my patients. The hospital has been on mask mandate for a little over two weeks now. At the hospital, it's scary, but rewarding at the same time. First and foremost, I want to thank everyone for your concern and help. The cards and food coming in from the community has been great in keeping morale and our spirits up.

The unit I work in is a COVID quarantine unit, the highest acuity and sickest patients we have in the health system. The patients' average age is in the fifties, but we have people who are in their twenties, thirties, forties, and fifties—much younger than we expected . . .

In the intensive care unit, one of many now throughout the hospital, we are using ventilators to help patients get enough oxygen. Under normal circumstances, not all ICU patients are on a vent. But right now with COVID-19, everyone in the ICU is on a breathing machine. This oxygen is helping them survive.

During the day, nurses come from all over to help us. Our nurse practitioner helps us monitor patients and gives us breaks. Everyone has come together to help. Our community is so important to us here. We just took the breathing tube out of one patient and are celebrating. We are all so excited. It was our second extubation of the day. It's great work.

Throughout the day, we need to take a deep breath and keep going on, powering through this unique situation. I'm on day five of doing thirteen-hour shifts. I'm tired. But I get to go home soon.

When I do get home, it's a little emotional. My nine-year-old daughter Eva usually runs and hugs me when I arrive. But we have social distancing now and she has to stay away until I properly decontaminate.

I don't bring anything into my house and have set up a decontamination station in my backyard. The kids bring the garbage out. We have a whole routine. My decontamination center includes Purell, Lysol wipes, and a garbage can. I make sure I wash my hands and take my scrubs off. I'm happy because I get to see my kids, but it's a little stressful because I can't yet hug them until after I shower . . .

Jeffrey Zilberstein, MD, is vice chair of medicine and director of Southside Hospital's intensive care units.
Working during COVID-19 has been challenging. I think that's the best way to put it. We keep getting more patients and since so many patients are very sick, they are having longer hospital stays. Given the number of patients we're seeing with the virus, we have opened the neuro ICU, surgical ICU, and cardiothoracic ICU to care for these patients. Each has a separate staff/team, although we are all working to care for COVID-19 patients together.

Given the large number of very sick patients that we're caring for, I am inspired by our staff every day and am seeing examples of us being "truly together" (one of our values) on a daily basis. They are willing to help any way they can, often "running into the fire" very willingly. Cardiologists and nephrologists, for instance, are helping me and my team care for our COVID-19 patients. I'm working with them in a capacity that makes the best use of their skills, supports the team, and ultimately helps our patients.

Every day is different for me. There are days when I'm able to see patients and then there are other days that it's more important for my team that I do more leadership-related tasks to support the staff and operations. Sometimes that feels like making organization out of chaos, but we always manage to do it, and I'm so proud of our team for doing that.

Southside Hospital is committed to making sure that our employees, especially those caring for COVID-19 patients, are taking the necessary time to rest and recharge. I make sure to not bother people on their off time whenever possible. I am also "calling in the cavalry" by obtaining resources from other Northwell locations or from the outside to relieve our staff whenever possible. Overall, our staff is resilient and I know that we will get through this.

When I come home from the hospital, I have stopped our family's usual practice of having the kids come hug me at the door, which is getting hard for them as time goes on. So we'll have to figure out how to manage that going forward. To prevent spreading germs to them, I make sure to change and take a shower before I speak to my family. I have also been trying to have playtime with my kids to help mentally keep myself going, although it has been hard to find time with the number of emails and things that need to be addressed after work hours. When I get home I sometimes feel part-human and part-android thanks to all the work emails.

I have been running for a while and meditating, both of which have been beneficial lately. The other day I ran on my treadmill with a monitor that made it look like I was running in Patagonia. That really helps to center me.

Bernard Robinson, EMT-P, is a regional director for Northwell Health's Center for Emergency Medical Services, overseeing daily operations of one of the largest EMS agencies on the East Coast.

The dramatic miniseries *Band of Brothers* details the bravery and fear shared among the members of the US Army's Easy Company, the 506th Regiment of the 101st Airborne Division in World War II. The company faced extraordinary circumstances, which called for extraordinary individuals and teamwork. Each carried another through seemingly insurmountable odds on D-Day and other battlefields.

As an emergency services worker on the front lines of the COVID-19 pandemic, I share the same camaraderie and uncertainties as those heroic men did so many years ago. There's a sense of pride within my unit. It doesn't matter who you are or where you came from, you are eager to volunteer, sacrificing yourself for the greater good and helping carry people through the illness.

When COVID's pace accelerated and overwhelmed New York, anxiety rose among the ranks of our staff, who were frantically dealing with regular calls and 911 calls and transferring patients out of the health system's hospitals to balance the load. At the height, we moved seventy-five to a hundred patients daily, which isn't surprising considering Northwell Health has treated more COVID-19 patients than any other health system in the United States. There were a lot of sleepless nights.

Then I became ill—a health scare like I've never had before, and I consider myself relatively healthy. Having COVID-19 curbed everything I knew of living, especially breathing. And despite being hospitalized for five days, afraid to sleep at times and now considered "recovered," I have reentered the battle against this deadly virus.

Why? Because working in emergency services is more than a profession. It's a calling. If my family—wife Connie and two boys, Elijah (twenty-one) and Christian (nineteen)—is my world, then my CEMS brothers and sisters are my oxygen. Returning to work was never a question in spite of my family's reservations . . .

I was exposed and unknowingly contracted the virus during a patient transport on Monday, March 23. Back then, I put aside my administrative duties as regional director to assist in the field. We covered overnight shifts to help facilitate transfers. There were a lot of sick patients, all of whom seemed to need to be ventilated.

For me, the coronavirus started as a dry cough. Nervousness immediately settled in, and four days later I tested positive. Literally every known symptom had emerged. The fatigue was the worst. Every two minutes I needed to sit still and catch my breath. COVID-19 was as debilitating as advertised.

Ultimately, I quarantined myself in my basement, away from my family and our typically busy household. I went to the hospital twice. After the first visit, I was diagnosed with pneumonia due to COVID-19 and was released. That night, I was extremely frightened, blowing through seven oxygen tanks just to breathe. I wasn't sure if I'd make it and refused to sleep.

My wife was nervous. My boys were scared. No one and no family should experience this.

The next day, I was admitted to North Shore University Hospital, where I stayed for five days, participated in a hydroxychloroquine clinical trial, and was treated with prednisone, oxygen, albuterol, and other medications. Breathing was my main issue, but it improved, and I was discharged on Easter morning—a blessing to watch a streaming service at my church before heading back to the basement. It was good to be home and feeling better, which is when I realized I needed to recover as fast as I could and get back to work.

That day came on Tuesday, April 21, just one month after testing positive. It's been slow progress. Toward the end of each day, my energy level tends to run down—the lingering effects of the virus. I'm immensely proud of the way our department has responded. Our team has protected themselves and helped thousands of people through this crisis, risking exposure during every COVID call.

I'm now mostly performing administrative duties and yearn to be back in the field . . . I'm still in uniform, though, and want to join everyone out there, ready for battle with my *Band of Brothers*.

Elisa Vicari, LCSW, is a social worker in the Intensive Care Unit at North Shore University Hospital.
As a social worker in the Intensive Care Unit at North Shore University Hospital, I've become immune to people passing away. Death is an unfortunate part of the job because we are treating the sickest patients.

COVID-19, though, was quite different for me and my colleagues.

During the patient surge in late March, we were caring for otherwise healthy twenty- and thirty-year-olds who were unaware of their surroundings and had no business being intubated. These are previously independent individuals who have been abruptly put on life support. This is the heartbreak the coronavirus leaves.

Adding to the complexities of this situation, visitation was restricted, and patients in our unit were unable to speak to their families. This didn't sit well, so I adapted my practice and refocused my efforts to find a solution. A quick Instagram post asking my friends and followers for one iPad donation turned into more than twenty and about eleven thousand dollars in community support—the true power of social media. Their assistance has allowed us to set up every unit within the hospital and other facilities in the area with iPads, which have been critical to helping us connect with families.

Not everyone is comfortable going into patient rooms. It's a personal choice that must be made, one that I did not struggle with. A social worker's role is to connect and assist, and the iPads have opened new roads to make important video calls where we could show not just a patient's condition, but the entire room and care team.

In the ICU, patients are mostly intubated. Finding close connections has been challenging. Instead, we have grown closer to families, FaceTiming with them every other day for status updates, learning nicknames and favorite songs, and hearing about their pets who await them at home. They've sent pictures so we can build collages and fill their rooms with love. I feel like I've become a part of these families just by holding the screen for them . . .

In some end-of-life circumstances, visitors have been allowed to see their loved ones in their final moments. We've been there to help them with PPE, addressing their fears and coping with their situation. Some are able to hold their family member's hand for the first time in weeks. We are also assisting with funeral arrangements, which are very different than usual with increased wait times. It's overwhelming, physically taxing, and mentally exhausting. But it's worth it. I couldn't imagine being on the other side, watching the terrible images on the news of beds with patients lined up and packed into places nearly on top of each other like wartime scenes. Showing families that our patients are in private rooms and we are helping them has given them tremendous comfort.

When patients fail, I feel it more than I used to because I've grown closer to them and their families. Our conversations aren't just based on medical concerns, but rather on vulnerable situations that I've now been welcomed into.

It's bittersweet. When things go well, they go well. But when they don't, it's devastating. At the heart of it, we deliver personalized, patient-centered, and compassionate care, pandemic or no pandemic. COVID-19 may have tested our mettle and capabilities, but we have survived thanks in part to the camaraderie between us and families. We have all met this challenge with innovation, compassion, and integrity. I really admire the people I work with who have stepped up. Teamwork is everything, knowing we will get through this together.

The angel of environmental services: *John Baez works in the Environmental Services Department at Staten Island University Hospital.*
In environmental services, we go above and beyond to make our patients feel comfortable and keep a clean environment. During COVID-19, we became their loved ones when their families couldn't be there and helped comfort them in their final moments. I've faithfully worked for Staten Island University Hospital for eleven years, and travel three hours each way from my home in Yonkers on public transportation to help care for patients.

I'm not a clinical care provider, but my dedication to patient safety in the Environmental Services (EVS) Department is what I strive for. My coworkers and I are at the top of our field when it comes to bedside manner and being spirited patient professionals. Unfortunately, our team is no stranger to a crisis. We saw the hospital through the evacuation ahead of Hurricane Irene, the aftermath from Superstorm Sandy the following year, and even the Ebola crisis in 2014.

But COVID-19 was something entirely different and something we never faced before. It put the EVS team on the front line to help contain and eliminate the virus, which tested all of our abilities. When the crisis was at its peak, I remember seeing one case after the other. People begging for their life, "I can't breathe, I can't breathe." Before coronavirus, I would always try to befriend and comfort the patients. During the crisis, I showed them love when their loved ones couldn't be at their bedside.

There was one day that would change me forever. It was a regular day, and then one of our patient care associates (PCAs) told me that this person is going to pass away. I knew the patient. I'd met her days earlier. It was the end of my shift and I was ready to take my first bus home, but I said to myself, "I can't let this woman pass alone. I'm going to be there for her."

I walked into the room and leaned over the patient and said, "It's me, John. If you hear me, squeeze my finger." She did. I told her, "I want you to go with God. I want you to relax and once you see the light, I want you to go to it. I'm going to hold your hand until you go."

The PCA cried alongside me. I told the patient I would pray for her. On her third breath, she passed. The doctor came in and checked her vitals, and confirmed what I already knew—she was gone.

I took the two buses and three trains home, replaying the day in my head. It's always going to be with me, the sadness that she couldn't have a loved one with her, but I couldn't let her die alone.

I did what many health-care heroes battling COVID-19 did: make the patients their second family and be their loved one. During this crisis, my mother was begging me to quit because we're dealing with something that's new and scary. But we all have to be here. It's our job. It's what we signed up for.

APPENDIX II

Recovery

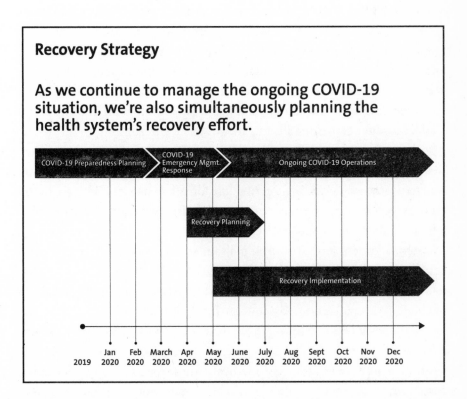

Recovery Strategy

As we continue to manage the ongoing COVID-19 situation, we're also simultaneously planning the health system's recovery effort.

COVID-19 Preparedness Planning

COVID-19 Emergency Mgmt. Response

Ongoing COVID-19 Operations

Recovery Planning

Recovery Implementation

| Jan 2020 | Feb 2020 | March 2020 | Apr 2020 | May 2020 | June 2020 | July 2020 | Aug 2020 | Sept 2020 | Oct 2020 | Nov 2020 | Dec 2020 |

2019

As complicated as the work had been to prepare for the onslaught of the coronavirus, the work to restore the Northwell system to some sort of normalcy would be, in the words of Mark Solazzo, "much more complex." But we shouldn't even use the term "normalcy," because that implies going back to the way things were. We have no intention of doing that. The world has changed and we have to change with it.

We are working our way through a series of questions including how, exactly, does this experience change the process of health-care delivery in the United States? How does it change the way consumers will want to access care? Will people be reluctant to go to the emergency department and prefer an urgent care center or a virtual visit? Certainly the convenience and effectiveness of telehealth was amply demonstrated during the crisis.

There are other questions we are wrestling with, as well, including: How should we at Northwell change internally? Should twenty thousand of our people continue to work from home? Do we need all the real estate—the office space and more—that we currently own or lease at great expense? This is not a time for normalcy or comfort. We have been pushed as never before as an organization. We not only were able to handle the crisis, but we actually emerged as a leader among our peers locally and nationally. If we get lazy and revert to the old normal we will lose an opportunity to revisit how we are organized and structured; to fix the inefficiencies and bureaucracy that we all know exist; to improve clinical care outcomes; to address inequities of care.

The recovery process will take a year at least, perhaps longer. Reopening is carefully regulated by the state. To complicate matters, our recovery process, including gearing up for a backlog of eighteen thousand surgeries, is taking place at the same time we are gearing up for a fall or winter surge in COVID cases.

Senior leaders started thinking about system recovery in April, well before the COVID peak in New York. Mark Solazzo gathered the directors of the three Northwell regions and explained that while we were managing the pandemic's assault on our hospitals, we would have to simultaneously begin thinking how we could get back to a place where it would be possible to take care of all of those people who had deferred treatment for a wide variety of medical issues. As each day of the crisis passed, more and more people needed treatment for other medical concerns. On April 14, a memo went out to leaders throughout the organization announcing that in the process of recovering from the pandemic, we would use the same incident command structure we used to prepare for it. Why was it so important to use this quasi-military command approach to get back to business? Because the incident command structure, when used properly, strips away bureaucracy and enables large organizations to behave in a flexible, innovative fashion. In a crisis, everything happens faster, and with the incident command approach, breaking normal organizational rules to get things done is a simple matter.

In preparing to start work toward recovery, Solazzo, as incident commander, made clear that he did not want to "go back to normal

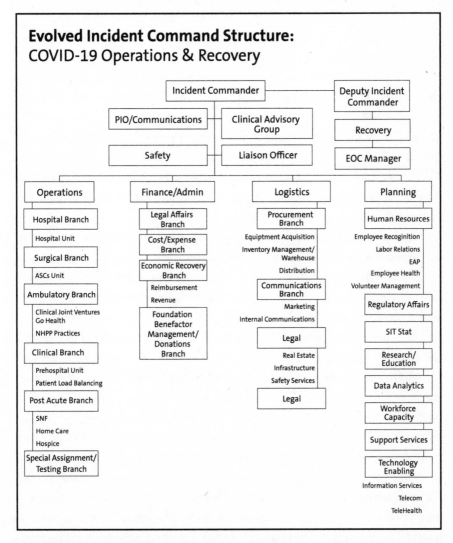

We evolved our original incident command structure to incorporate all of the new developed recovery work streams.

operations." Rather, he sought to take advantage of lessons learned in the crisis "and change our organization for the better."

Change is hard and many people in medicine are reflexively change-averse. But change on a widespread basis would be more doable under the incident command structure where thoughtful action was prized over lengthy deliberation and soul-searching. Operating under incident command allows you to "maintain a focused effort of analysis, very quick consensus-building, and decision-making," said Solazzo. "It shortens the timeline from problem to decision to execution." We needed to sacrifice a certain amount of consensus for speed so that we could change our organization quickly. Solazzo estimated that, working at a normal pace, it would take eighteen months to recover, but by doing it at speed under the incident command structure, we could do it in six. "You try to build consensus as much as possible, but it is not as democratic," he said. "We want everybody on the same train, but we're not going to wait until everybody gets on because we don't have the luxury of time to do that. This event had a very, very significant operational and financial impact on this organization that we need to correct in order to maintain the vision and the mission that we hold dear."

And to pursue our mission we have to make sure that we are able to safely care for the enormous pent-up demand for services that built during the crisis. We started the recovery by having our clinical leaders prioritize which surgeries are most urgent and which can wait until a bit later. These physicians came up with a series of guidelines that ensured safety. In order to demonstrate to patients and staff that we could safely restart the surgery program, we set up our hospital at Syosset as a model. All COVID patients were transferred from Syosset to other facilities. Then the hospital was deep cleaned and sanitized. The staff is fully equipped with PPE, and patients arriving in the parking area are greeted by a valet who provides them with a mask, and then they are escorted directly to a treatment room, bypassing the waiting area. Every visible sign is designed to assure patients that the environment is safe. All surgical patients must self-quarantine for fourteen days and then, twenty-four to forty-eight hours prior to the procedure, we test them for the virus. Then they return to quarantine until the operation. On the day of surgery everybody entering the hospital is screened with a thermal screener and then assessed for possible symptoms. We also want patients to understand that we have always safely taken care of patients with highly contagious conditions. Protecting staff and other patients from contagions is a skill that is essential to any major health system's ability to function effectively.

In April, as Solazzo began to contemplate how to go about the work of recovery, he developed twelve project work streams, each of which was to be led by a senior leader and supported by teams of experienced individuals. The project work streams are:

Hospital operations: Ensure that our hospitals are able to transition to recovery while managing the ongoing crisis, and to optimize the use of our facilities into the "New Normal." This group sought answers to questions like: What do you do to prevent crowded elevators? Do you allow visitors back in to see patients? Perhaps one visitor at a time? Do you require visitors to wear PPE? Going forward, all of our hospitals will include a mix of patients—some with COVID, many with a variety of other ailments. The crucial point here is that we have learned a great deal about how to isolate COVID patients so that they—and everyone else in the hospital—are safe. "We are able to create separation as soon as they hit our doors and maintain that separation throughout the patient's stay," said Solazzo.

Surgical operations: Plan for the reintroduction of all of our surgical services. This involves the basic work of taking back the perioperative spaces that were used as temporary ICUs, cleaning and reconstituting the anesthesia machines, and making certain they are safe for use in operations. It also involves giving the staff members who were moved from surgical services to frontline roles time off so they can be refreshed when coming back to work.

Ambulatory operations: Prepare our ambulatory network to reopen as rationally, efficiently, and quickly as possible. In the New Normal, we envision our ambulatory sites working in partnership with virtual health to accommodate patients and doctors in whatever way best serves the patient. A difficult aspect of this is reassessing our need for as many ambulatory sites as we had and deciding on possible closures. This team made progress early in establishing how to create a safe environment within our ambulatory locations with Plexiglas partitions in some areas, instituting just-in-time arrivals, and establishing plenty of space in waiting areas for social distancing.

Clinical operations: Ensure alignment of our clinical resources across the continuum to provide the safest, most efficient patient experience possible. The essential question here is: How do you make sure that you bring the patient in to the right location? We were inspired by the load-balancing work done during the crisis when patients were sent to the places where there was the right staff and equipment to care for them. The idea of applying this to normal clinical operations is very appealing. For example, let's say a patient is in the hospital and has been treated successfully. Rather than going through the often cumbersome and bureaucratic discharge process, what if we applied a central load-balancing capability to what happens next to that patient? What if that central load-balancing function had the ability and authority to select the right next step for the patient—a rehab facility, nursing home, or skilled nursing facility—and then do all the work needed to secure a placement and transport the patient to the new location? And then could the load-balancing case manager arrange for follow-up home visits for the patient as well as a videoconference with the pulmonologist the following week? "We want to take the administrative load off of the nurse and the physician on the floor, letting them focus on their clinical activity," said Solazzo, by having the central logistics center arrange everything—all the authorizations that need to occur with the insurance agencies, transportation, appointments that need to be scheduled, and home care with a respiratory therapist or a physical therapist. Said Solazzo: "We're building this as a twenty-four hour a day, seven days a week operation, and we think it will make us much more efficient."

COVID-19 resurgence operations: Continued vigilance against an unpredictable virus and planning for possible resurgence into the foreseeable future. As we have noted earlier in the book, this crisis was different from our experiences in the past with hurricanes, blackouts, and other events that happen in a short period of time and then are over. While we are recovering, we must remain vigilant for a possible COVID-19 recurrence or for another malevolent virus that finds its way to our area. What do we need to be doing now for a second wave? How big do we think the second wave is going to be? Our current estimate is that it could be larger than the first wave. Dr. Wayne Breining is very concerned about the virus recurring in the winter of 2021: "We have to identify people for symptoms as soon as possible. We can do random testing to see who picks up the virus and identify anybody who may have been exposed to them, anybody who may be the source of their infection, and you can use fairly standard isolation and quarantine procedures to limit the spread of the infection whenever you see it emerging."

Clinical advisory: Provide insight and support to ensure that safe, high-quality care is delivered throughout the recovery period and beyond. This massive responsibility involves input on every decision with any medical implications at all, which means virtually every decision we make.

Support services: Ensure that our support services remain mobilized to support frontline operations while planning for a sustainable future. This includes all central office services, including finance, IT, HR, and purchasing. To say the least, it was a revelation that we were able to function effectively as an organization when suddenly, without any warning, twenty thousand staff members from support services were required to work remotely. It worked so well that we found that many employees increased their efficiency. We extended the remote work through the summer and will decide later which functions can continue on a work-from-home basis and which really do need to be in the office. Or perhaps there is a hybrid in some area—three days in the office, two days at home. It gets slightly complicated: What HR structures do we put in place to make that workforce still feel like part of our culture? How do we bring them in on occasion? How do we make certain that they have career pathways, and that we're recognizing them? "It's not just about handing somebody a computer and saying, do your work at home," said Solazzo. "We would lose the culture that we worked so hard to create here. How do you keep them motivated and passionate about the work? Remote work also opens us up to a much larger labor pool. Work doesn't have to be done in a specific town, or within a thirty-mile commute. Work can be done globally now, and it could be both globally and locally, or domestically or foreign. It gives us opportunities and flexibility."

Technology leverage: Advance the use of our clinical technology platforms to assist in maximizing patient and clinician access. Technology (or lack thereof) is a constant complaint of everyone in health care, especially those at the bedside. The goal of this group is not only to work with the system's Chief Information Officer John Bosco and to rethink the pre-COVID list of technology priorities, but also to take advantage of the exciting innovation that occurred during the response and to have the ability to fast-track many IT innovations. An example is technology we deployed throughout the hospitals to keep families connected to their loved ones and to the care teams. Within one week we were able to automate sending test results to patients via text message or email and to use our "list app" application to inform the call center when the patient acknowledged receipt of the results electronically.

Communications: Maintain our pipeline of information to our workforce and to our communities while establishing new messaging on a safe and sustainable recovery. The goal here is to communicate to the public that we are fully open and can care for whatever health needs anyone in our communities happens to have.

Financial stability: Create a road map to financial stability through revenue recovery opportunities and greater system-wide efficiencies. It is very expensive to go through the process of recovering a huge health system, and we have to make sure that we have the cash available to do whatever we need to, while at the same time getting us back to the position of financial stability we enjoyed before anyone had ever heard of COVID-19.

Employee recognition and resilience: Take the lead in creating the work plan to celebrate the heroic efforts of our workforce and to provide support to them as they move forward from this crisis. This area is of enormous importance. Our employees lifted up our organization, and we owe them everything. We have paid bonuses to every frontline worker despite the organization being in the red by a billion dollars. We have set up funds to support families of our employees who passed away during the crisis. We gave every frontline worker an extra week of paid vacation. But there is much more to be done. We are watching carefully for signs of burnout or psychological effects from the crisis. Maureen White, chief nursing executive, is particularly attuned to the psychological needs of staff members. She witnessed the response of nurses whose team members had died, and these survivors, she said, suffered a terrible sense of loss, even depression. She worries about an emergence in some staff members of trauma well after the fact, not unlike the psychological issues that people face after combat.

APPENDIX III

Key Metrics and Key Milestones

Key Metrics

COVID-19 Daily Dashboard Metrics

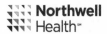

Below is a summary of daily metrics followed throughout the COVID crisis along with a definition of each metric.

THROUGHPUT	
Total Acute Care Beds On Site	Total number of acute care beds in the hospital. (Excludes OB, Psych, Rehab, etc. unless activated as an inpatient unit under the hospital's surge plan)
ICU Beds On Site	Total number of ICU beds in-house, inclusive of converted units associated with the ICU surge plan
ICU Occupancy	(ICU Beds: In Use) / (ICU Beds: Available)
Current patients in isolation	Number of patients with isolation orders or isolation status sent from registration at a point in time
Total Patients on All Vents	Patients on vents + Patients on anesthesia machines being used as vents + All patients on BiPAP V60
Total COVID+ Patients on All Vents	COVID+ pts on vent + Patients on anesthesia machines being used as vents + BiPAP V60 used invasively in COVID+ patients
Vents on Site	Number of ventilators on site (Excludes Anesthesia machines being used as vents)
Vents Available	(Vents On-Site) - (Patients on Vents)
Vent Capacity (% of Vents in Use)	Patients on Vent divided by the number of Vents On-Site
Patients on Mechanical Vent	Number of patients on a ventilator (Excludes anesthesia machines being used as vents)
Anesthesia Machines Being Used as Vents	Number of anesthesia machines converted to Vents (not included in the "Vents on Site" number)
Patients on Anesthesia Machines Being Used as Vents	Number of patients on anesthesia machines converted to vents (not included in the "Patients on Vents" number)
Anesthesia Machines Left for Surgery	Total number of anesthesia machines on-site, less anesthesia machines coverted to vents
BiPAP V60 used invasively in Non COVID pts	BiPAP V60 used invasively in Non COVID pts (used on ET/Trach Pts)
BiPAP V60 used invasively in COVID Positive pts	BiPAP V60 used invasively in COVID Positive patients
BiPAP V60 used non-invasively	BiPAP V60 used non-invasively (via a mask for sleep apnea, post extubation support etc.)
BiPAP V60 available	Total BiPAP V60 on site minus (Invasive BiPAP Non-COVID positive patients + Invasive BiPAP COVID positive patients + Non-Invasive BiPAP)
Available Morgue Capacity	(Standard Morgue Capacity + Additional Surge Morgue Capacity) - Number of Morgue Spaces Occupied
EMERGENCY DEPARTMENT	
3 Hr ER Door to Provider (min)	The average number of minutes a patient waited to see a doctor over the past 3 hours (minutes from quick reg until provider enters room)
ER Holds	The raw number of patients with ED disposition = ADMIT who have not yet left the ED for their destination

COVID-19 Daily Dashboard Metrics

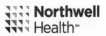

Below is a summary of daily metrics followed throughout the COVID crisis along with a definition of each metric.

COVID-19 STATUS	
In-House COVID-19 Tests Ordered	The raw number of patients currently admitted who have a non-cancelled COVID-19 PCR (or equivalent) order
In-House COVID-19 Tests Pending	The raw number of patients currently admitted who have a non-cancelled COVID-19 PCR (or equivalent) order and results are still pending
In-House COVID Positive Patients	The raw number of patients currently admitted who have a non-cancelled COVID-19 PCR (or equivalent) order and resulted in positive
COVID Patients in ICU (%)	(COVID positive in ICU) / (In-House COVID Positive Patients)
COVID Patients on Vent (%)	(COVID positive on Vent) / (In-House COVID Positive Patients)
Discharges to SNF On Hold	Number of COVID+ patients ready to be discharged to SNF and put on hold
Prior Day COVID+ Discharges	The raw number of COVID-19 positive patients discharged yesterday (includes deaths). For prepopulated sites, this is the time of discharge in sunrise equal to yesterday.
Prior Day COVID+ Mortality	The raw number of COVID-19 positive patients expired yesterday (discharge status = Expired). For prepopulated sites, this is the time of discharge in sunrise equal to yesterday.
Prior Day Covid Negative Admissions	The raw number of COVID-19 negative patients admitted to the inpatient unit yesterday. Patient was admitted through the emergency department.
Prior Day No Test Admissions	The raw number of patients admitted to the inpatient unit yesterday, with no COVID-19 test result. Patient was admitted through the emergency department.

Key Milestones

Northwell Health™

Novel Coronavirus (COVID-19) Event 2020 NYS Key Milestones

February

- 2/1 – NYS DOH designates COVID-19 as a communicable disease, requiring reporting, etc.
- 2/3 – NYS DOH provides update for healthcare providers on COVID-19, including a review of reporting and testing requirements, screening for illness, PPE recommendations, etc.
- 2/6 – NYS DOH issues recommendations to hospitals regarding PPE, CDC guidelines, potential for PPE shortages, process for requesting state assistance.
- 2/11 – NYS DOH issues a Notice to Healthcare Providers regarding persons at risk for COVID-19 who present for medical care (isolation, PPE, etc.).
- 2/14 – NYS DOH issues COVID-19 guidance to EMS practitioners, county emergency managers, county EMS coordinators.
- 2/20 – NYS DOH begins weekly COVID-19 updates to healthcare providers.
- 2/25 – Governor Cuomo directs New Yorkers who have returned from China since February 3 to voluntarily quarantine.
- 2/26 – Governor Cuomo pledges $40 million to fight the virus, asks federal authorities to allow the state's Wadsworth Center to test for COVID, proposes legislation to grant the Governor broad authority to suspend laws in a crisis. Announces DOH convening local health departments and hospitals throughout the state to review protocols, procedures, best practices.
- 2/28 – Governor Cuomo receives federal approval to begin COVID testing at the Wadsworth Center.

March

- 3/1 – Governor announces state's first case of COVID-19, confirmed by Wadsworth Center, the state's public health laboratory.
- 3/2 – Legislature passes Governor's Bill to appropriate $40m and to give him extraordinary powers.
- 3/2 – Governor Cuomo announces plan for Wadsworth Center to partner with hospitals to expand COVID testing; announces a new cleaning protocol for use in schools and the public transportation system.
- 3/2 – Governor announces that NYS DFS will direct health insurers to waive cost sharing for COVID testing, including emergency room, urgent care, and office visits; announces promulgation of emergency regulations; and issues additional guidance to insurers regarding COVID.
- 3/3 – Governor signs legislation authorizing $40m emergency management authorization for COVID response; SUNY institutions recalling students from study-abroad programs.

*For a summary of all executive orders, refer to document provided by Legal Department (#149366)

Novel Coronavirus (COVID-19) Event 2020 NYS Key Milestones

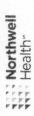
Northwell
Health™

March

- 3/3 – Governor announces state's second case of COVID-19.
- 3/4 – Governor announces four new cases of COVID-19 in Westchester County; outlines protocols to minimize potential spread in the area.
- 3/5 – Governor announces additional COVID cases downstate; activates the statewide Emergency Operation Center and satellite centers; announces federal approval for state to work with hospital labs at Northwell Health and SUNY Stony Brook to expand COVID testing.
- 3/6 – Governor announces additional COVID cases; announces the NYS Interagency COVID Task Force is coordinating efforts of local governments and healthcare providers.
- 3/7 – Governor issues Executive Order 202, declaring a disaster emergency in the state resulting from an outbreak of COVID-19. This EO also temporarily suspended and modified laws to expedite the state's abilities and authorities to respond to the outbreak. https://www.governor.ny.gov/news/no-202-declaring-disaster-emergency-state-new-york
- 3/9 – NYS DOH issues interim guidance for COVID-19 testing and for containment, quarantine, and isolation.
- 3/10 – Governor directs implementation of containment plan in New Rochelle, including partnership with Northwell Health for the state's first drive-through testing site.
- 3/10 – NYS DOH issues recommendations to protect nursing home residents.
- 3/11 – Governor announces contract with 28 private laboratories to expand COVID testing capacity; demands FDA approval.
- 3/11 – NYS DOH issues COVID-19 guidance to nursing homes and adult care facilities.
- 3/12 – Governor announces limitations on mass gatherings.
- 3/12 – Governor issues Executive Order 202.1. https://www.governor.ny.gov/news/no-2021-continuing-temporary-suspension-and-modification-laws-relating-disaster-emergency
- 3/13 – NYS DOH issues COVID-19 guidance for large gatherings and public spaces, requiring cancellations and limitations.
- 3/13 – NYS receives FDA authority to conduct COVID testing at public and private laboratories.
- 3/14 – Governor issues Executive Order 202.2. https://www.governor.ny.gov/news/no-2022-continuing-temporary-suspension-and-modification-laws-relating-disaster-emergency
- 3/14 – NYS DOH issues COVID-19 guidance to home health agencies, long-term home health care programs, hospices, and licensed home care agencies.

*For a summary of all executive orders, refer to document provided by Legal Department (#149366)

Novel Coronavirus (COVID-19) Event 2020 NYS Key Milestones

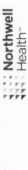

Northwell Health

March

- 3/15 – Governor announces closure of New York City, Westchester, Suffolk and Nassau schools.
- 3/16 – Governor announces a regional coalition of the states of New York, New Jersey and Connecticut to coordinate COVID actions to reduce the spread of the virus, including limitations on gathers, closures of restaurants, bars, gyms, casinos, and movie theaters.
- 3/16 – Governor issues Executive Order 202.3. https://www.governor.ny.gov/news/no-2023-continuing-temporary-suspension-and-modification-laws-relating-disaster-emergency
- 3/16 – Governor issues Executive Order 202.4. https://www.governor.ny.gov/news/no-2024-continuing-temporary-suspension-and-modification-laws-relating-disaster-emergency
- 3/16 – NYS DFS announces a special, extended enrollment period for uninsured New Yorkers to enroll through NY State of Health and insurers to obtain coverage in light of COVID.
- 3/16 – NYS DOH issues COVID-19 guidance to home care programs.
- 3/17 – Governor announces agreement with the Legislature on Paid Sick Leave to provide immediate assistance to those impacted by COVID.
- 3/17 – NYS DFS adopts emergency regulation requiring insurers to waive cost-sharing for in-network telehealth services.
- 3/17 – NYS DOH requires immediate suspension of adult care facilities day programs for non-residents.
- 3/18 – Governor announces deployment of hospital ship USNS Comfort to New York City.
- 3/18 – Governor issues Executive Order 202.5. https://www.governor.ny.gov/news/no-2025-continuing-temporary-suspension-and-modification-laws-relating-disaster-emergency
- 3/18 – Governor issues Executive Order 202.6. https://www.governor.ny.gov/news/no-2026-continuing-temporary-suspension-and-modification-laws-relating-disaster-emergency
- 3/18 – NYS DOH issues COVID-19 guidance restricting hospital visitation.
- 3/18 – NYS DOH issues process for emergency approvals for COVID-19 surge capacity for hospitals and diagnostic & treatment centers.
- 3/18 – NYS DOH issues COVID guidance for Community Based Long-Term Services and Supports covered by Medicaid.
- 3/18 – Governor announces that Pennsylvania is joining the NY, NJ, CT, regional coalition.
- 3/19 – Governor issues Executive Order 202.7. https://www.governor.ny.gov/news/no-2027-continuing-temporary-suspension-and-modification-laws-relating-disaster-emergency
- 3/19 – NYS DOH issues COVID-19 guidance for Children and Family Treatment and Support Services' providers.

Page 3|8

*For a summary of all executive orders, refer to document provided by Legal Department (#149366)

Novel Coronavirus (COVID-19) Event 2020 NYS Key Milestones

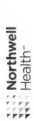
Northwell
Health™

March

- 3/19 – NYS DOH issues COVID guidance for Facilitated Enrollment Agencies for the aged, blind, and disabled.
- 3/20 – Governor signs "New York State on PAUSE".
- 3/20 – Governor announces multi-state regional coalition coordinating the closure of barber shops, hair and nail salons, and related services.
- 3/20 – Governor issues Executive Order 202.8. https://www.governor.ny.gov/news/no-2028-continuing-temporary-suspension-and-modification-laws-relating-disaster-emergency
- 3/20 – NYS DFS issues guidance to insurers to suspend pre-authorization and administration requirements such as utilization review to facilitate hospital immediate treatment of COVID patients.
- 3/20- NYS DOH issues nursing home advisory for recommendations to protect nursing home residents.
- 3/20 – NYS DOH issues guidance for Nursing Home Transition and Diversion, and Traumatic Brain Injury Medicaid Waiver providers.
- 3/21 – Governor announces sites for temporary surge hospitals in cooperation with the Army Corps of Engineers.
- 3/21 – Governor issues Executive Order 202.9. https://www.governor.ny.gov/news/no-2029-continuing-temporary-suspension-and-modification-laws-relating-disaster-emergency
- 3/21 – NYS DOH issues guidance for pregnancy and COVID-19.
- 3/21 – NYS DOH issues a Health Advisory to nursing homes and adult care facilities regarding presumptive COVID-19 cases in New York City, Long Island, and Westchester and Rockland Counties.
- 3/21 – NYS DOH issues guidance for nursing homes seeking emergency approval to provide home hemodialysis services to residents.
- 3/22 – NYS DOH issues guidance to adult care facility operations regarding PPE and other issues.
- 3/22 – NYS DOH issues guidance to home health care agencies and hospice providers regarding COVID-19 screening of patients and staff.
- 3/22 – NYS DOH issues COVID-19 guidance for dental health care settings, including postponement of non-essential dental care.
- 3/23 – Governor issues Executive Order 202.10. https://www.governor.ny.gov/news/no-20210-continuing-temporary-suspension-and-modification-laws-relating-disaster-emergency
- 3/23, 4/4, 4/29 – NYS DOH issues guidance to hospitals regarding non-essential, non-urgent elective surgeries and procedures.
- 3/23 – NYS DOH applies to the federal government for a COVID-19 Medicaid 1135 Waiver.

*For a summary of all executive orders, refer to document provided by Legal Department (#149366)

Novel Coronavirus (COVID-19) Event 2020 NYS Key Milestones

Northwell Health™

March

- 3/24 – NYS DFS adopts emergency regulation requiring regulated financial institutions to provide relief to those demonstrating financial hardship as a result of the COVID outbreak, including forbearance of payment, elimination of ATM fees, credit card late payment fees, etc.
- 3/25 – NYS DOH issues guidance for specimen collection and handling for COVID-19 testing.
- 3/26 – NYS DOH conducts webinar on COVID-19 infection control guidance for nursing homes and adult care facilities.
- 3/27 – Governor announces the readiness of 1,000 bed temporary hospital at the Jacob K. Javits Convention Center.
- 3/27 – Governor issues Executive Order 202.11. https://www.governor.ny.gov/news/no-20211-continuing-temporary-suspension-and-modification-laws-relating-disaster-emergency
- 3/28 – Governor issues Executive Order 202.12. https://www.governor.ny.gov/news/no-20212-continuing-temporary-suspension-and-modification-laws-relating-disaster-emergency
- 3/28 – NYS DOH issues a Health Advisory on recommendations for release of individuals from home isolation.
- 3/30 – Governor issues Executive Order 202.13. https://www.governor.ny.gov/news/no-20213-continuing-temporary-suspension-and-modification-laws-relating-disaster-emergency
- 3/31 – NYS DOH issues protocols for essential personnel returning to work following COVID-19 exposure or infection.

April

- 4/2 – Governor announces NYS DOH approval of Northwell Health protocol to convert BiPAP machines to ventilators.
- 4/2 – NYS DOH issues a Health Advisory to all healthcare providers regarding options when PPE is in short supply or unavailable.
- 4/2 – NYS DFS announces emergency regulation allowing consumers and businesses to defer payment of individual and small group commercial health insurance premiums through June 1 as a result of financial hardships from the COVID outbreak.
- 4/4 – NYS DOH issues guidance for resident and family communication protocols in adult care facilities and nursing homes.
- 4/5 – Governor announces federal government is deploying 1,000 medical personnel to New York State.
- 4/7 – Governor issues Executive Order 202.14. https://www.governor.ny.gov/news/no-20214-continuing-temporary-suspension-and-modification-laws-relating-disaster-emergency

*For a summary of all executive orders, refer to document provided by Legal Department (#149366)

Novel Coronavirus (COVID-19) Event 2020 NYS Key Milestones

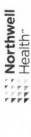

April

- 4/7 – NYS DOH issues an advisory mandating that all adult care facilities have a process in place to expedite return of asymptomatic residents from the hospital, and clarifying that no resident shall be denied admission or re-admission based on a confirmed or suspected diagnosis of COVID-19.

- 4/8 – NYS DOH issues a Health Advisory on COVID-19 and the use of cloth face coverings.

- 4/9 – Governor issues Executive Order 202.15. https://www.governor.ny.gov/news/no-20215-continuing-temporary-suspension-and-modification-laws-relating-disaster-emergency

- 4/10 – Governor announces ramp up of COVID antibody testing as part of a plan to prepare to reopen the economy.

- 4/10 – NYS DOH issues COVID infection prevention and control preparedness checklist and self-assessment for long-term care facilities.

- 4/10 – NYS DOH issues guidance on regulatory relief in home health agencies, long term home health care programs, licensed home care agencies, AIDS home care programs, and hospices.

- 4/10 – NYS DOH issues guidance for home health aide training programs.

- 4/10 – NYS DOH issues updated COVID guidance for funeral directors.

- 4/10 – NYS DOH issues updated COVID guidance suspending all hospital visitation with exceptions for patients in imminent end-of-life situations.

- 4/12 – Governor announces he is requiring employers to provide cloth or surgical masks to essential employees who interact with the public.

- 4/12 – Governor issues Executive Order 202.16. https://www.governor.ny.gov/news/no-20216-continuing-temporary-suspension-and-modification-laws-relating-disaster-emergency

- 4/13 – Governor announces creation of a multi-state council with NY, NJ, CT, PA, DE, RI to coordinate plans to restore the economy.

- 4/15 – Governor announces requirement that all people wear masks or face coverings in public.

- 4/15 – Governor issues Executive Order 202.17. https://www.governor.ny.gov/news/no-20217-continuing-temporary-suspension-and-modification-laws-relating-disaster-emergency

- 4/16 – Governor issues Executive Order 202.18. https://www.governor.ny.gov/news/no-20218-continuing-temporary-suspension-and-modification-laws-relating-disaster-emergency

- 4/17 – Governor issues Executive Order 202.19. https://www.governor.ny.gov/news/no-20219-continuing-temporary-suspension-and-modification-laws-relating-disaster-emergency

- 4/18 – Governor calls for federal coordination of supply chain to bring COVID testing to scale.

- 4/18 – Governor issues Executive Order 202.20. https://www.governor.ny.gov/news/no-20220-continuing-temporary-suspension-and-modification-laws-relating-disaster-emergency

:::Northwell
:::Health™

Page 6 | 8

*For a summary of all executive orders, refer to document provided by Legal Department (#149366)

Novel Coronavirus (COVID-19) Event 2020 NYS Key Milestones

April

- 4/19 – Governor issues Executive Order 202.21. https://www.governor.ny.gov/news/no-20221-continuing-temporary-suspension-and-modification-laws-relating-disaster-emergency
- 4/19 – NYS DOH issues guidance to nursing homes regarding management of resident deaths during the COVID outbreak.
- 4/19 – NYS DOH issues guidance to private physician practices regarding large-scale specimen collection sites for COVID testing.
- 4/19 – NYS DOH issues a Health Advisory regarding discontinuation of isolation for patients with COVID.
- 4/19 – NYS DOH issues guidance on resident and family communication in adult care facilities and nursing homes.
- 4/20 – Governor issues Executive Order 202.22. https://www.governor.ny.gov/news/no-20222-continuing-temporary-suspension-and-modification-laws-relating-disaster-emergency
- 4/21 – Governor announces elective outpatient surgery can resume in counties and hospitals which meet NYS DOH criteria.
- 4/22 – Governor announces partnership with Bloomberg Philanthropies to build a COVID contact tracing program to control COVID infection rate.
- 4/22 – NYS DFS issues guidance to health insurers to provide cash flow relief to, and ease administrative burdens on, hospitals.
- 4/23 – Governor announces partnership of NYS DOH and State Attorney General to investigate nursing home violations.
- 4/24 – Governor issues Executive Order 202.23. https://www.governor.ny.gov/news/no-20223-continuing-temporary-suspension-and-modification-laws-relating-disaster-emergency
- 4/25 – Governor announces expansion of COVID diagnostic testing to include all first responders, health care workers, and essential employees.
- 4/25 – Governor issues Executive Order 202.24. https://www.governor.ny.gov/news/no-20224-continuing-temporary-suspension-and-modification-laws-relating-disaster-emergency
- 4/29 – Governor issues Executive Order 202.25. https://www.governor.ny.gov/news/no-20225-continuing-temporary-suspension-and-modification-laws-relating-disaster-emergency
- 4/29 – Governor announces 35 counties approved to resume elective outpatient surgeries and procedures.
- 4/29 – Governor accepts recommendations from the COVID Maternity Task Force.
- 4/30 – Governor and Mayor announce MTA plans daily disinfection of NYC Transit System.
- 4/30 – NYS DOH issues guidance to clinical and other laboratories regarding reporting of COVID results.
- 4/30 – NYS DOH issues guidance on COVID serology testing.

Northwell Health

*For a summary of all executive orders, refer to document provided by Legal Department (#149366)

Northwell Health™

Novel Coronavirus (COVID-19) Event 2020 NYS Key Milestones

May

- 5/1 – Governor announces all schools and college facilities statewide will remain closed for the rest of the academic year.
- 5/1 – Governor issues Executive Order 202.26. https://www.governor.ny.gov/news/no-20226-continuing-temporary-suspension-and-modification-laws-relating-disaster-emergency
- 5/2 – Governor announces results on ongoing antibody testing study.
- 5/2 – NYS DFS issues emergency regulations requiring insurance companies to waive out-of-pocket costs for in-network mental health services for frontline essential workers during the COVID outbreak.
- 5/3 – Governor announces multi-state coalition will develop regional supply chain for supplies.
- 5/4 – Governor outlines additional guidelines for when regions can re-open.
- 5/5 – Governor issues Executive Order 202.27. https://www.governor.ny.gov/news/no-20227-continuing-temporary-suspension-and-modification-laws-relating-disaster-emergency
- 5/7 – Governor issues Executive Order 202.28. https://www.governor.ny.gov/news/no-20228-continuing-temporary-suspension-and-modification-laws-relating-disaster-emergency
- 5/8 – Governor announces NYS DOH is investigating COVID-related severe illness in children.
- 5/8 – Governor issues Executive Order 202.29. https://www.governor.ny.gov/news/no-20229-continuing-temporary-suspension-and-modification-laws-relating-disaster-emergency
- 5/9 – Governor announces initiative to expand access to testing in low-income communities and communities of color in partnership with Northwell Health.
- 5/9-10 – Governor announces that NYS DOH is helping to develop national criteria for identifying and responding to COVID-related illness in children, and is notifying 49 other states of the occurrence of this illness.
- 5/10 – Governor issues Executive Order 202.30. https://www.governor.ny.gov/news/no-20230-continuing-temporary-suspension-and-modification-laws-relating-disaster-emergency
- 5/11 – Governor announces three regions of the state are ready to begin reopening May 15.
- 5/12 – Governor directs hospitals to prioritize COVID testing for children.
- 5/13 – Governor announces NYS DOH to hold statewide webinar for healthcare providers to discuss inflammatory disease in children related to COVID.

*For a summary of all executive orders, refer to document provided by Legal Department (#149366)

Acknowledgments

We are grateful to many of our colleagues here at Northwell for their stories and insights. Our appreciation goes to Dr. Teresa Amato, Susan Browning, John Bosco, Steve Bello, Kevin Beiner, Adam Boll, Dr. Wayne Breining, Maria Carney, Dr. James Crawford, Michelle Cusack, Dr. Martin Doerfler,

Donna Drummond, Jeanne Gabriel, Sven Gierlinger, Howard Gold, Matt Jelavic, Holly Koehler, James Kostolni, Jeff Kraut, Jason Philip, Brian Lally, Terry Lynam, Mary Mahoney, Phyllis McCready, Rita Mercieca, Joe Moscola, Karen Nelson, Brian O'Neill, Curtis Reisinger, Shane Sabert, Dr. Ankita Sager, Tom Sclafani, Jon Sendach, Merryl Siegel, Ramon Soto, Alex Trinkoff, Lee Weisman, and Dennis Whalen.

At Skyhorse Publishing we are indebted to Tony Lyons, Caroline Russomanno, and Brian Peterson.

The two leaders of our Incident Command structure, Mark Solazzo and Gene Tangney, provided important insight and guidance. Our executive nursing leader Maureen White was particularly insightful. And our physician advisors—Drs. Mark Jarrett, John D'Angelo, David Battinelli, Kevin Tracey, Lawrence Smith, Debbie Salas-Lopez, and Thomas McGinn—were invaluable in helping us understand various aspects of the disease and its treatments.